The **Juice Lady's**

BIG BOOK of JUICES & Green Smoothies

The **Juice Lady's**

BIG BOOK
of JUICES
& Green
Smoothies

Cherie Calbom, MS, CN

SILOAM

Most CHARISMA HOUSE BOOK GROUP products are available at special quantity discounts for bulk purchase for sales promotions, premiums, fund-raising, and educational needs. For details, write Charisma House Book Group, 600 Rinehart Road, Lake Mary, Florida 32746, or telephone (407) 333-0600.

THE JUICE LADY'S BIG BOOK OF JUICES AND GREEN SMOOTHIES by Cherie Calbom
Published by Siloam
Charisma Media/Charisma House Book Group
600 Rinehart Road
Lake Mary, Florida 32746
www.charismahouse.com

Cover design by Justin Evans
Design Director: Bill Johnson

Visit the author's website at www.cheriecalbom.com.

Library of Congress Cataloging-in-Publication Data
Calbom, Cherie.
   The juice lady's big book of juices and green smoothies : more than 400 simple, delicious recipes! / Cherie Calbom. -- First edition.
        pages cm
   Summary: "Juices and smoothies are sweeping the nation because of their nutritional benefits. This book gives benefits of the various ingredients used in vegetable and fruit juicing, plus 400 recipes to put these benefits to use in great-tasting juices and smoothies, with specifics for different physical conditions"-- Provided by publisher.
   Includes bibliographical references.
   ISBN 978-1-62136-030-8 (pbk.) -- ISBN 978-1-62136-031-5 (ebook) (print)
   1. Smoothies (Beverages)--Therapeutic use. 2. Fruit juices--Therapeutic use. I. Title.
   RM237.C25 2013
   615.3'21--dc23
                                        2012035292

13 14 15 16 17 — 9 8 7 6 5 4 3 2
Printed in the United States of America

CONTENTS

INTRODUCTION

ORE AND MORE celebrities, athletes, and people of all ages and walks of life are turning to juicing and green smoothies to lose weight and to improve their overall health. Why? Because they have found that juicing is changing their lives—giving them more energy, better sleep, stronger immune systems, brighter skin, and a younger appearance. It's even helping their bodies heal from a variety of ailments. Below is a testimony I received recently from someone who has read my books and come to me for counseling.

It's been about a month since you last spoke with me. You may not remember me because you talk with so many people. But I will never forget you. I told you about the more than fifty pounds of fluid I had retained. Using both natural and medical prescriptions, I had not been able to get rid of that fluid. I have also not been absorbing my food. You told me not to worry about my diet because I already had a healthy one but to add a green juice drink with every meal. About three weeks before I spoke with you I started drinking pure cranberry juice every day, and that was helping with the fluid. Over the three weeks I lost fifteen pounds, but I would bounce back and forth with my weight. When I added the green juice drinks, it put my body in high gear. I have lost thirty pounds. The water weight is literally just falling off of me.

You have no idea how much better I am feeling. I have energy and can physically work. I have not had energy or felt good since my last baby was born twenty-five years ago. I have not been able to push my body to work for the last five years. Now I am splitting firewood and stacking it. I shoveled rock for our drainage system in our yard. I can clean my own house again. Yesterday I cleaned house and stacked two cords of firewood. If you haven't stacked firewood, let me tell you, that's a lot of wood. And I can walk again. For the last two years I have been fighting just to walk up and down my short driveway, feeling totally exhausted and in pain afterward. Now I am easily walking a mile and have energy to burn. I feel great and have no pain when I'm finished. And my fibromyalgia pain is almost gone.

For the last five years I have been fighting to stay alive. Now for the first time in years I feel *alive*. I am no longer on Lasix and have cut back most of my nutritional supplements. I was taking over $500 worth of supplements a month, and it was bankrupting us. Last year my doctor told me to apply for disability because my body was dying. I could no longer function. The naturopathic physician I used to work for told me that my husband and I needed to accept the fact that my body was dying. He told us to purchase better health insurance and prepare for the worst. I wish he could see me now.

Long story short, Cherie, I am so grateful to you for taking the time to talk with me. I know you probably hear stories like mine all the time, but for me it's new and life saving. Thanks for pointing me to the path of life. You have been one of God's blessings and a lifesaver in the most literal sense of the word.

I hope her story encourages you to juice every day. With more than four hundred delicious recipes, *The Big Book of Juices and Green Smoothies* can help you change your life, just as juicing has changed the lives of thousands of people who have adopted this plan for themselves—people just like me. My life changed years ago when I discovered the healing, vitality-producing power of freshly made juices and raw and whole foods.

Sick, Tired, and Completely Toxic

I sat by the window in my father's home in Colorado staring at the snow-topped mountains in the distance, imagining that people were enjoying the hiking trails; perhaps someone was climbing the mountain that day. It was early June and a beautiful, sunny Colorado day. I wished I had the strength to just walk around the block. But I was too sick and tired—I could barely walk around the house. I had been sick for a couple of years and just kept getting worse. "Would I ever be well again?" I wondered.

I had to quit my job when I turned thirty. I had chronic fatigue syndrome and fibromyalgia that made me so sick I couldn't work. I felt as though I had a flu that just wouldn't go away. I was lethargic and constantly feverish with swollen glands. I was also in nonstop pain. My body ached as though I'd been bounced around in a washing machine.

I had moved back to my father's home in Colorado to try and recover, but not one doctor could tell me what I should do to improve my health. So I browsed around some health food stores, talked with employees, and read a few books. I decided that everything I'd been doing was tearing down my health rather than healing my body. When I read about juicing and whole foods, it made sense. So I bought a juicer and designed a program I could follow.

I began my health program with a five-day vegetable juice fast. On the fifth day my body expelled a tumor the size of a golf ball. I was totally surprised that in five days this amazing result could take place. I never did have the tumor tested because I was too taken back and overwhelmed by the event. I just flushed it away.

I then continued to juice every day and ate a nearly perfect diet of live and whole foods for three months. There were ups and downs throughout. On some days I felt encouraged that I was making some progress, but on other days I felt worse. Those days made me wonder if good health was an elusive dream. I didn't realize I was experiencing detox reactions—no one had told me about them. I was very toxic, and my body was cleansing away all the stuff that had made me sick.

But one morning I woke up around 8:00 a.m., which was early for me, without an alarm sounding off. I felt like someone had given me a new body in the night. I had so much energy I actually wanted to exercise. What had happened? This new feeling of good health and vitality had just appeared with the morning sun. Actually, my body had been healing all along; it just had not manifested fully until that day. I felt such a wonderful sense of being alive! I looked and felt completely renewed.

With my juicer in tow and a new lifestyle fully embraced, I returned to Southern California and my friends a couple weeks later to finish writing my first book. For nearly a year it was "ten steps forward" with great health and more energy and stamina than I'd ever remembered. Then all of a sudden I took a giant step back.

The Night I'll Never Forget

The Fourth of July was a beautiful day like so many others in Southern California. I celebrated the holiday with friends at a backyard barbecue. That evening we put on jackets to insulate against the cool evening air and watched fireworks light up the night sky. I returned just before midnight to the house I was sitting for vacationing friends, who lived in a lovely neighborhood not far from some of my family members. After such a full day I was in bed shortly after I arrived at the house.

I woke up shivering some time later wondering why it was so cold. I rolled over to see the clock. It was 3:00 a.m. That's when I noticed that the door was open to the backyard. "How did that happen?" I thought as I was about to get up to close and lock the door. That's when I saw him. Crouched in the shadows of the corner of the room was a shirtless young man in shorts. I blinked twice, trying to deny what I was seeing.

Instead of running out the open door, he leaped off the floor and ran toward me. He pulled a pipe from his shorts and began beating me repeatedly over the head and yelling, "Now you are dead!" We fought, or I should say, I tried to defend myself and grab the pipe. Finally it flew out of his hands. That's when he choked me to unconsciousness. I felt all life leaving my body. In those last few seconds I knew I was dying. "This is it, the end of my life," I thought. I felt sad for the people who loved me. Then I felt my spirit leave. It felt as though it just popped out of my body and floated upward. Suddenly everything was peaceful and still. I sensed I was traveling through black space at what seemed like the speed of light. I saw what looked like lights twinkling in the distance.

But all of a sudden I was back in my body, outside the house, clinging to a fence at the end of the dog run. I don't know how I got there. I screamed for help with all the energy I had. It was my third scream that took all my strength. I felt it would be my last breath. Each time I screamed, I passed out and landed on the cement. I then had to pull myself up again. But this time a neighbor heard me and sent her husband to help. Before long I was on my way to the hospital.

Lying on a cold gurney at 4:30 a.m., chilled to the bone, in and out of consciousness, I tried to assess my injuries, which was virtually impossible. When I looked at my right hand, I almost passed out again. My ring finger was hanging on by a small piece of skin. My hand was split open, and I could see deep inside. The next thing I knew I was being wheeled off to surgery. Later I learned that I had suffered serious injuries to my head, neck, back, and right hand, with multiple head wounds and part of my scalp torn from my head. I also incurred numerous cracked teeth, which led to several root canals and crowns months later.

My right hand sustained the most severe injuries. Two of my knuckles were crushed to mere bone fragments and had to be held together with three metal pins. Several months after the attack I still couldn't use my hand. The cast I wore, which had bands holding up the ring finger that had almost been torn from my hand and various odd-shaped molded parts, looked like something from a science-fiction movie. I felt and looked worse than hopeless. The top of my head was shaved, and my eyes were totally red and swollen. I had a gash on my face, a weird-looking right hand, terrorizing fear, and barely enough energy to get dressed in the morning.

I was an emotional wreck. I couldn't sleep at night—not even a minute. It was torturous. I was staying with a cousin and his family, so there was no need to worry about safety from a practical point of view, but that made no difference to me emotionally. I'd lie in bed all night and stare at the ceiling or the bedroom door. I had five lights that I kept on all night. I'd try to read, but my eyes would sting. I could sleep only for a little while during the day.

But the worst part was the pain in my soul that nearly took my breath away. All the emotional pain of the attack joined with the pain and trauma of my past to create an emotional tsunami. My past had been riddled with loss, trauma, and anxiety. My brother died when I was two. My mother died of cancer when I was six. I couldn't remember much about her death—the memories seemed blocked. But my cousin said I fainted at her funeral. That told me a lot.

I lived for the next three years with my maternal grandparents and father. But Grandpa John, the love of my life, died when I was nine. That loss was very hard. Four years later my father was involved in a very tragic situation that would take far too long to discuss here, but to sum it up—it was horrific. He was no longer in my daily life. I felt terrified about my future. My grandmother was eighty-six. I had no idea how much longer she would live. The next year I moved to Oregon to live with an aunt and uncle until I graduated from high school.

As you can probably imagine, wrapped in my soul was a huge amount of anguish and pain—it felt like gaping holes in my heart. It took every ounce of my will, faith, and trust in God; deep spiritual work; alternative medical help; extra vitamins and minerals; vegetable juicing; emotional release; healing prayer; and numerous detox programs to heal physically, mentally, and emotionally. I met a nutritionally minded physician who had healed his own slow-mending broken bones with lots of vitamin-mineral IVs. He gave me similar IVs. Juicing, cleansing, nutritional supplements, a nearly perfect diet, prayer, and physical therapy helped my bones and other injuries heal.

After following this regimen for about six months, what my hand surgeon said would be impossible became real. My hand was fully restored and fully functional. He had told me I'd never use my right hand again, and that it wasn't even possible to implant plastic knuckles because of its poor condition. But my knuckles did indeed re-form primarily through prayer, and my hand function returned. A day came when the surgeon told me I was completely healed, and though he admitted he didn't believe in miracles, he said, "You're the closest thing I've seen to one."

It was a miracle! I had a useful right hand again, and my career in writing was not over as I thought it would be. In the end it seemed my inner wounds were the most severe and the hardest to heal. Nevertheless, they mended too. I experienced healing from the painful memories and trauma of the attack and the wounds from the past through prayer, laying-on of hands, and deep emotional healing work.

I call them the *kitchen angels*—the ladies who prayed for me around their kitchen tables week after week until my soul was restored. It seemed I cried endless buckets of tears that had been pent up in my soul. It all needed release. Forgiveness and letting go came in stages and was an integral part of my total healing. I had to be honest about what I really felt and be willing to face the pain and toxic emotions confined inside, and then let them go. Finally, one day after a long, long journey—I felt free. A time came when I could celebrate the Fourth of July without fear.

A New Beginning

When I look back to that first day in the hospital after many hours of surgery, it's amazing to me that I made it. My hand was resting in a sling hanging above my head. It was wrapped with so much stuff it looked like George Foreman's boxing glove. My face had a big cut running down the left side, and my eyes were red—very little whites. A maintenance man came into my room for a repair and did a double take. He asked if I'd been hit by a truck! He was serious. I felt like I had. As I lay there alone with tears streaming down my face, I asked God if He could bring something good out of this horror. I needed something to hang on to.

My prayer was answered. Eventually I knew my purpose was to love people to life through my writing, juicing, and nutritional information— to help them find their way to health and healing. If I could recover from all that had happened to me, they could too. No matter what anyone faced, there was hope.

Juice Recipes for Health and Healing

In the pages that follow, you'll discover a wide variety of juices for every possible need and occasion. I have basic juice recipes for those who are getting started and want something simple. There are yummy fruit juice recipes for those with picky palates who want the sweet taste of fruit. Green juices are my favorite and offer the most nutrition; you'll find a big selection of green juice recipes to choose from.

Check out the chapter on juice remedies and rejuvenators for juice combos that address what ails you. And I think you'll really like the gourmet juice chapter that has a lot of unique combinations and delicious drinks. There's also the green smoothie chapter with one hundred smoothie recipes and great combinations. And I also included my old favorites from *The Juice Lady's Turbo Diet* and *The Juice Lady's Living Foods Revolution*. Have fun trying some new and unusual combinations. There's a lot to choose from with more than four hundred recipes.

And if you're struggling with your health, there is hope for you, no matter what health challenges you face. Never, ever give up. There's a purpose for your life, just as there was for mine. You need to be healthy and strong to complete your purpose. To that end, *The Juice Lady's Big Book of Juices and Green Smoothies* can help you live your life to the fullest. My hope is that this book of delicious recipes will truly inspire you to juice each and every day and that you will experience firsthand the healing, rejuvenating power of fresh juice and green smoothies.

Chapter 1

ALL ABOUT JUICING

WHETHER YOU ARE just getting started juicing or you've been juicing a long time, you probably have a few questions about this subject. In this chapter I answer most of the questions I am frequently asked about juicing and juice nutrition. I also share guidelines for choosing a good juicer. And I answer some frequently asked questions about making juice, such as which fruits and vegetables should be peeled first and which seeds can be juiced. I also give you plenty of tips to make juicing easy and fun.

How many times have you eaten a meal and not long after felt tired, lethargic, or spacey? Obviously, based on your body's reaction, that was not a good food choice. Yet how often do we keep eating the same things over and over again, even though they don't help us feel better, more energized, or more alert? If you want good health, eat foods that love you back. Fresh juices, especially fresh veggie juices, will love you back all the time by giving you energy, vitality, and better mental performance.

I hope to inspire you to make juicing a daily habit. It can change your life, just as it changed Marie's. Here's her story:

Last year I took a huge leap of faith and opened my own business—a running store. I have been a runner for thirty years, and for the past eleven of those years I have been a running coach and manager of a running store. I experienced many early mornings lying wide-awake in bed wondering what I was doing. I was twenty pounds heavier than when I started my running career and had a bad back—not a good combination when you're a marathon-training coach. My physical condition did not help the stress level I was experiencing trying to get a new business off the ground. I was at a breaking point and didn't even know it.

I mentioned to some friends that I wasn't feeling well. That was all it took. Along came my angels—although at first I did not see them as such. Two friends whom I respect asked me to do a ten-day juice cleanse with them. Um, that would be a *no*. First, I really like my glass of wine at night, and cooking is my way of relaxing. I like my lattes in the morning, and on it went. My list of excuses was rather long—there were a lot of "reasons" I was not interested. I ended by telling them that these kinds of things never work. Being the quiet angels they are, they didn't push or try to talk to me into it. But the next morning I arrived at work to find *The Juice Lady's Turbo Diet* book by Cherie Calbom sitting on my desk. I pushed it aside. I had way too much to do. But for some reason, that night I put it in my bag. Was there an unseen angel at work?

When I awoke at 2:00 a.m. unable to fall back to sleep, I wanted something to read. And there it was—*The Juice Lady's Turbo Diet*. I read that book until the sun came up. Everything Cherie talked about resonated. Believe me when I say I have tried everything. I have done everything from no carbs (not a good plan for endurance athletes) to the eating plan I was on at the time, which was living on energy bars during the day and coming home at night and throwing all the good nutrition advice I gave my runners out the window as I ate everything in sight because I was starving.

Everything Cherie explained, I started to understand,

such as when your body does not process your food properly, it is unable to utilize the nutrients properly. Instead of your food acting as fuel, what you eat turns into fat. And the body needs to be cleansed periodically or the toxins keep you from losing the fat. The light bulb went on! I realized my organs were not processing very well the food I was eating.

I was now intrigued. I wanted to eliminate the foods Cherie suggested in the Turbo Diet and follow her diet plan of juicing and eating clean. I was determined to eliminate dairy, gluten, and animal protein to see if I felt a difference. I did a three-day cleanse and was on *fire*! I was losing weight, and my energy level was increasing.

Then I watched *Fat, Sick and Nearly Dead*, and the one who said, "I would never do a ten-day juice cleanse," was so excited to do a ten-day cleanse I rushed out and bought Cherie's book *Juicing, Fasting and Detoxing for Life*. I bought a better juicer and tons of produce. Game on.

I was so excited to see how my body would feel and even more intrigued by the emotional detoxing Cherie's book said might take place. Everything she described in the juicing, fasting, detox book was true. I lost all my cravings. I wasn't hungry. After day three on her program I completely stopped thinking about food. At the end of one month, with a three-day cleanse, clean eating, and a ten-day juice feast (I like calling it that more than fast), I was twelve pounds lighter. (To date, I've lost twenty pounds.) And better yet, I was back to my happy and energetic self.

People coming into the store have noticed the changes— my skin is brighter and, of course, I'm leaner. And people say I look younger. My juice revolution was on. If I could do this, anyone could. I was on a mission with all my newfound energy

Why Is Juice So Effective in Changing Lives?

Every time you pour a glass of juice, picture a big vitamin-mineral cocktail with a wealth of nutrients that promote vitality. The veggies are broken down into an easily absorbable form that your body can use—right away. This food doesn't have to go through a big process of breaking everything down. So it goes to work in your body to give you energy and renew you right down to your cells. It also spares your organs all the work it takes to digest food, and that equates to more energy. It detoxifies your body as well because it's rich in antioxidants, so that lightens your load, and the body doesn't have to work so hard to deal with all the toxic stuff.

The Nutritional Components of Fresh Juice

In addition to water and easily absorbed protein and carbohydrates, juice also provides essential fatty acids, vitamins, minerals, enzymes, biophotons, and phytonutrients. And researchers are continuing to explore how the nutrients found in juice help the body heal and shed unwanted pounds. The next time you make a glass of fresh juice, this is what you'll be drinking:

Protein

When you think of protein sources, does juice ever come to mind? Probably not, but surprisingly it does offer more than you might think. We use protein to form muscles, ligaments, tendons, hair, nails, and skin. Protein is needed to create enzymes, which direct chemical reactions, and hormones, which guide bodily functions. Fruits and vegetables contain lower quantities of protein than animal foods such as muscle meats and dairy products. Therefore they are thought of as poor protein sources. But juices are concentrated forms of vegetables and fruit and so provide easily absorbed amino acids, the building blocks that make up protein. For example, 16 ounces of carrot juice (2 to 3 pounds of carrots) provides about 5 grams of protein (the equivalent of about one chicken wing or 2 ounces of tofu). Vegetable protein is not complete protein, so it does not provide all the amino acids your body needs. In addition to lots of dark leafy greens, you'll want to eat other protein sources, such as sprouts, legumes (beans, lentils, and split peas), nuts, seeds, and whole grains. If you're not vegan, you can add eggs and free-range, grass-fed muscle meats such as chicken, turkey, lamb, and beef along with wild caught fish.

Carbohydrates

Vegetable and fruit juices contain carbohydrates. Carbs provide fuel for the body, which uses it for movement, heat production, and chemical reactions. The chemical bonds of carbohydrates lock in the energy a plant takes up from the sun, and this energy is released when the body burns plant food as fuel. There are three categories of carbs: simple (sugars), complex (starches and fiber), and fiber. Choose more complex carbohydrates than simple carbs in your diet. There are more simple sugars in fruit juice than vegetable juice, which is why you should juice more vegetables and in most cases drink no more than 4 ounces of fruit juice a day. Both insoluble and soluble fibers are found in whole fruits and vegetables, and both types are needed for good health. Who said juice doesn't have fiber? Juice has the soluble form—pectin and gums, which are excellent for the digestive tract. Soluble fiber also helps to lower blood cholesterol levels, stabilize blood sugar, and improve good bowel bacteria.

Essential fatty acids

There is very little fat in fruit and vegetable juices, but the fats juice does contain are essential to your health. The essential fatty acids (EFAs)—linoleic and alpha-linolenic acids in particular—found in fresh juice function as components of nerve cells, cellular membranes, and hormonelike substances called prostaglandins. They are also required for energy production.

Vitamins

Fresh juice is loaded with vitamins. Vitamins take part, along with minerals and enzymes, in chemical reactions. For example, vitamin C participates in the production of collagen, one of the main types of protein found in the body. Fresh juices are excellent sources of water-soluble vitamins such as C; many of the B vitamins and some fat-soluble vitamins such as vitamin E; the carotenes, known as provitamin A (they are converted to vitamin A as needed by the body); and vitamin K. They also come packaged with cofactors, such as vitamin C with bioflavonoids. The cofactors and vitamins help each other be more effective.

Minerals

Fresh juice is loaded with minerals. There are about two dozen minerals that your body needs to function well. Minerals, along with vitamins, are components of enzymes. They make up part of bones, teeth, and blood tissue, and they help maintain normal cellular function. The major minerals include calcium, chloride, magnesium, phosphorus, potassium, sodium, and sulfur. Trace minerals are those needed in very small amounts, which include boron, chromium, cobalt, copper, fluoride, manganese, nickel, selenium, vanadium, and zinc. Minerals occur in inorganic forms in the soil, and plants incorporate them into their tissues. As a part of this process, the minerals are combined with organic molecules into easily absorbable forms, which make plant food an excellent dietary source of minerals. Juicing is believed to provide even better mineral absorption than whole vegetables because the process of juicing liberates minerals into a highly absorbable, easily digestible form.

Enzymes

Fresh juices are chock-full of enzymes—those "living" molecules that work with vitamins and minerals to speed up reactions necessary for vital functions in the body. Without enzymes we would not have life in our cells. Enzymes are prevalent in raw foods, but heat such as cooking and pasteurization destroys them. All juices that are bottled, even if kept in store refrigerators, have to be pasteurized. Heat temperatures for pasteurization are required to be far above the limit of what would preserve the enzymes and vitamins.

When you eat and drink enzyme-rich foods, these little proteins help break down food in the digestive tract, thereby sparing the pancreas, small intestine, gallbladder, and stomach—the body's enzyme producers—from overwork. This sparing action is known as the "law of adaptive secretion of digestive enzymes." According to this law, when a portion of the food you eat is digested by enzymes present in the food, the body will secrete less of its own enzymes. This allows the body's energy to be shifted from digestion to other functions such as repair and rejuvenation. Fresh juices require very little energy expenditure to digest, and that is one reason people who start consistently drinking fresh juice often report that they feel better and more energized right away.

Phytochemicals

Plants contain substances that protect them from disease, injury, and pollution. These substances are known as phytochemicals. *Phyto* means "plant," and *chemical* in this context means "nutrient." There are tens of thousands of phytochemicals in the foods we eat. For example, the average tomato may contain up to ten thousand different types of phytochemicals, the most famous being lycopene. Phytochemicals give plants their color, odor, and flavor. Unlike vitamins and enzymes, they are heat stable and can withstand cooking. Researchers have found that people who eat the most fruits and vegetables, which are the best sources of phytochemicals, have the lowest incidence of cancer and other diseases. Drinking vegetable juices gives you these vital substances in a concentrated form.

Biophotons

There's one more substance, more difficult to measure than the others, that's present in raw foods. It's being studied scientifically in tubes and is named biophotons. It's light energy that the plants absorb from the sun, and it is found in the living cells of raw foods such as fruits and vegetables. Photons have been shown to emit coherent light energy when uniquely photographed (using Kirlian photography). This light energy is believed to have many benefits when consumed; one in particular is thought to aid cellular communication. Biophotons feed the mitochondria of the cells, which produce ATP—our body's energy fuel. Biophotons are also believed to contribute to our energy, vitality, and a feeling of vibrancy and well-being.

Frequently Asked Questions

Now that you know why juice is so effective for good health, you may have some questions about juicing. Below I will address some of the questions I am most commonly asked about juicing.

Why juice? Why not just eat the fruits and vegetables?

Though I always tell people to eat their vegetables and fruit, there are at least three reasons juice is important and should also be included in the diet. First, we can juice far more produce than we would probably eat in a day. It takes a long time to chew raw veggies. Chewing is a very good thing. I highly encourage it. However, we have only so much time for chewing raw foods. One day I timed how long it would take for me to eat five medium-size carrots. (That's what I often juice along with cucumber, lemon, ginger root, beet, kale, and celery.) It was about fifty minutes of chewing. Not only do I not have that kind of time every day, my jaw was so tired afterward that I could hardly move it.

LIGHT AFFECTS NUTRIENTS

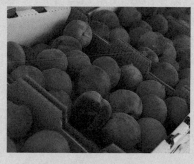

Do you select your produce from the front of a display, or do you reach to the back, hoping you'll find the ones that are freshest and least picked over? If you think the hidden produce is the best, a new study may convince you to choose your fruits and veggies differently. Scientists from the US Department of Agriculture (USDA) recommend that consumers select their produce from those receiving the greatest light—usually the ones found at the front or top of the display. For example, researchers found that spinach exposed to continuous light during storage was more nutritionally dense than spinach that was continually in the dark. The scientists said light affects the leaves' photosynthetic system, which resulted in an increase in vitamins C, E, K, and folate.[1]

Secondly, we can juice parts of the plant we would not normally eat, such as stems, leaves, and seeds. I juice things I know I would rarely or never eat, such as beet stems and leaves, celery leaves, the white pithy part of the lemon with the seeds, asparagus stems, broccoli stems, the base of cauliflower, kohlrabi leaves, radish leaves, and ribs of kale.

Thirdly, juice is broken down so it spares digestion. It is estimated that juice is at work in the system in about twenty to thirty minutes after it is consumed. When we have ailments, juice is therapy for this very reason. When the body has to work hard to break down veggies, for example, it can spend a lot of energy on the digestive process. Juicing does the work for you. So when you drink a glass of fresh juice, all those life-giving nutrients can go to work right away to heal and repair your body, giving it energy for its work of rejuvenation.

Don't we need the fiber that's lost in juicing?

It's true that we need to eat whole vegetables, fruit, sprouts, legumes, and whole grains for fiber. We drink juice for the extra nutrients; it's better than any vitamin pill. And for weight loss I recommend vegetable juices for appetite control. I also recommend juice as therapy. I cover more than fifty different ailments in my book *The Juice Lady's Guide to Juicing for Health* that can be improved with juice therapy, diet, and nutrients. Whole fruits and vegetables have insoluble and soluble fiber. Both types of fiber are very important for colon health. It's true that the insoluble fiber is lost when you juice. However, soluble fiber is present in juice in the form of gums and pectins. Soluble fiber is excellent for the digestive tract. It also helps to lower blood cholesterol, stabilize blood sugar, and improve good bowel bacteria. Don't worry about the fiber that is lost when you juice. Think about all the extra nutrition you are getting. Fresh juice is one of the best vitamin-mineral cocktails you could drink. You may not need as many nutritional supplements when you juice, so that could save you money in the long run. Drink your juice as a smart addition to your high-fiber diet.

Are a lot of nutrients lost with the fiber?

In the past some groups have thought that a significant amount of nutrients remained in the fiber after juicing, but that theory has been disproved. The US Department of Agriculture analyzed twelve fruits and found that 90 percent of the antioxidant nutrients they measured was in the juice rather than the fiber.[2] This makes fresh juice a great supplement in the diet.

Is fresh juice better than commercially processed juice?

Fresh juice is "live food" with a full complement of vitamins, minerals, phytochemicals, and enzymes. It also contains biophotons that revitalize the body. You feel better when you drink fresh juice! In contrast, commercially processed canned, bottled, frozen, or packaged juices have been pasteurized, which means the juice has been heated and many of the vitamins and enzymes have been killed or removed. And the light energy is virtually gone. If you look at a Kirlian photograph of a cooked vegetable or a pasteurized glass of juice, you'll see very little "light" or no light emanating from them. This means the juice will have a longer shelf life, but it won't give your body life. Making your own juice also allows you to use a wider variety of vegetables and fruit you might not otherwise eat, such as kale, beets with leaves and stems, lemon with the white part, stems, seeds, and chunks of ginger root. Some of my recipes include Jerusalem artichokes, jicama, green cabbage, celery leaves, asparagus stems, broccoli stems, kale, and parsley. These sweet, crisp tubers and healthy greens are not found in most processed juices.

How long can fresh juice be stored?

The sooner you drink fresh juice after you make it, the more nutrients you'll get. However, you can store juice and not lose too many nutrients by keeping it cold in an insulated container or covered in the refrigerator. You can also freeze it. Many busy moms are choosing to make a large batch of juice on the weekends and freeze it in individual containers.

On a personal note, when I had chronic fatigue syndrome, I would juice in the afternoons when I had the most energy and store the juice covered in the refrigerator and drink it for the next twenty-four hours until I juiced my next batch. I got well doing that.

How much produce is needed to make a glass of juice?

People often ask me if it takes a basket of produce to make a glass of juice. Actually, if you're using a good juicer, it takes a surprisingly small amount. For example, the following items yield about one 8-ounce glass of juice: five to seven large carrots or one large cucumber. The following each yield about 4 ounces of juice: one large apple, three to four large (13-inch) ribs of celery, or one large orange. The key is to get a good juicer that yields a dry pulp. I've used juicers, even expensive models, that ejected very wet pulp. When I ran the pulp through the juicer again, I got more juice and the pulp was still wet. If the rotation speed (RPM) is too high or the juicer is not efficient in other ways, you will waste a lot of produce.

Will juicing cost a lot of money?

If you were to crunch the numbers, you would find that the cost of a glass of juice is less than a latte. With three or four carrots, half a lemon, a chunk of ginger root, two ribs of celery, three or four green leaves, and half a cucumber, you will probably spend two dollars to three and a half dollars, depending on the season, the area of the country you live in, and the store where you purchase your produce. But wait—there are also hidden savings. You may not need as many vitamin supplements. What's that worth? And you'll probably need far fewer over-the-counter medications such as painkillers; sleeping aids; antacids; and cold, cough, and flu medications. That's a whopping savings! And then there's time not lost from work. What happens when you run out of sick days? Or if you're self-employed, you've missed out on income each day you're sick. With the immune-building, disease-fighting properties of fresh juice, you should stay well all year long.

HOW TO CHOOSE THE RIGHT JUICER

Choosing the right juicer can make the difference between juicing daily and never juicing again, so it's important to get one that works for your lifestyle. I'm often asked if a blender can be used instead of a juicer, and unfortunately you can't use a blender to make juice, no matter how high-powered or expensive it is. A juicer separates the liquid from the pulp (insoluble fiber). A blender liquefies everything that is placed in it; it doesn't separate the insoluble fiber from the juice. If you think it might be a good idea to have carrot, beet, parsley, and celery pulp in your juice for added fiber, I can tell you from experience that it tastes like juicy mush. For the best juice, which is juice you'll enjoy and drink every day, you need a juicer. These are the features you should look for:

- Choose a machine with *adequate horsepower* (hp). I recommend a juicer with 0.3 to 1 hp. Weak-motored machines with low horsepower ratings must run at extremely high RPM (revolutions per minute). However, a machine's RPM does not accurately reflect its ability to perform effectively, because RPM is calculated 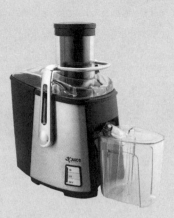 when the juicer is running idle, not while it is juicing. When you feed produce into a low-power machine, the RPM will be reduced dramatically, and sometimes the juicer will come to a full stop. I have "killed" some machines on the first carrot I juiced.

- Make sure the juicer is *efficient at extracting juice*. I've used a number of juicers that wasted a lot of produce because there was a lot of juice left in the pulp. You should not be able to squeeze a lot of juice out of the pulp. Some machines have an RPM that is too high, and the pulp comes out very wet. I've had people tell me they were spending a lot of money on produce and getting only a small amount of juice, which should not be the case. It often turned out that they were wasting a lot of produce because of an inefficient juicer.

- Look for a machine that has *electronic circuitry* that sustains blade speed during juicing.

- The juicer *should be able to juice all types of produce*. Make sure the machine can juice tough, hard vegetables, such as carrots and beets, as well as delicate greens, such as parsley, lettuce, and herbs. Make sure it doesn't need a special citrus attachment. For wheatgrass juice, you'll need a wheatgrass juicer or a juicer that presses the juice, such as a single auger or twin gear machine, also known as a masticating juicer. Be aware that the machines that juice wheatgrass along with other vegetables and fruit take more time to use. Some are more time consuming to clean as well.

- Look for a *large feed tube* if you don't have a lot of time to devote to juicing. Cutting your produce into small pieces before juicing does take time. A large feed tube will allow you to juice more quickly. Be aware that the masticating style juicers have small openings at the top, so you will need to spend a little more time preparing your produce.

- Look for a juicer with *only a few parts to clean*. The more parts a juicer has, and the more complicated the parts are to wash, the longer it will take to clean up and the more time it will take to put it back together. That makes it less likely you will use your machine daily. Also make sure the parts are dishwasher-safe. It's very easy to just rinse the parts and let them air dry. It really helps to spray the blade basket if you have a separate faucet sprayer. This can blow out fiber particles very quickly. Then take a soft-bristle dish brush and brush both sides quickly under running water. I clean the lid, blade basket, and juice bowl in this manner in less than a minute.

Two Types of Juicers: Centrifugal and Masticating

The centrifugal, or centrifuge, juicers typically have an upright design. Food is pushed into a rapidly spinning mesh blade basket with sharp teeth. The teeth shred the produce into a pulp, and the centrifugal motion pulls the juice out of the pulp and through the mesh filter, where it is funneled out of the juicer via a spigot and the pulp is ejected into a catcher. Centrifugal juicers will not juice wheatgrass. Another drawback is that the juice will not last as long as juice made with a masticating type of juicer because more oxygen is incorporated into the juice. There is also some indication that there are fewer nutrients in juice from centrifugal devices due to the extracting process of the juicer.

The masticating type of juicer produces juice with either a single auger or twin gear. Pieces of fruits and vegetables are fed into the top of the tube and are crushed and squeezed. Juice drains out of the underside, while the pulp is pushed out at the end of the tube. Because of the slower crushing and squeezing action, masticating juicers can process wheatgrass and will juice leafy greens a little better than a centrifugal juicer. The juice these devices produce will last much longer than juice made in a centrifugal juicer, and there is indication that more nutrients are preserved. The drawbacks are that they take longer to make juice because they are slower, and produce has to be cut in smaller pieces because they do not come with wide mouths.

Which one is the best type of juicer? The one you will use every day.

The Basics of Juicing

Juicing is a very simple process. Simple as the procedure is, though, it helps to keep a few guidelines in mind to obtain the best results.

- *Wash all produce before juicing.* Fruit and vegetable washes are available at many grocery and health food stores. Or you can use hydrogen peroxide and then rinse. Cut away all moldy, bruised, or damaged areas of the produce.

- *Always peel oranges, tangerines, tangelos, and grape-fruit* before juicing, because the skins of these citrus fruit contain volatile oils that can cause digestive problems such as stomachaches. Lemon and lime peels can be juiced, if organic, but they do add a distinct flavor that is not one of my favorites for most recipes. I usually peel them. Leave as much of the white pithy part on the citrus fruit as possible, though, since it contains the most vitamin C and bioflavonoids. Bioflavonoids work with vitamin C; they need each other to create the best uptake for your immune cells. Always peel mangoes and papayas since their skins contain an irritant that is harmful when eaten in quantity.

I also recommend that you peel all produce that is not labeled organic even though the largest concentration of nutrients is in and next to the skin. For example, nonorganic cucumbers are often waxed, trapping the pesticides. You don't want the wax or pesticides in your juice. The peels and skins of sprayed fruits and vegetables contain the largest concentration of pesticides.

- *Remove pits, stones, and hard seeds* from fruits such as peaches, plums, apricots, cherries, and mangoes. Softer seeds from cucumbers, oranges, lemons, limes, watermelons, cantaloupes, grapes, papaya, and apples can be juiced without a problem. Because of their chemical composition, large quantities of apple seeds should not be juiced for young children under the age of two, but they should not cause problems for older children and adults.

- *The stems and leaves of most produce can be juiced.* Beet stems and leaves, strawberry caps, celery leaves, radish leaves, and small grape stems are all fine to juice, and they offer nutrients. Discard larger grape stems, as they can dull the juicer blade. Also remove carrot tops and rhubarb greens because they contain toxic substances. Cut off the ends of carrots since this is the part that molds first.

- *Cut fruits and vegetables into sections or chunks* that will fit into your juicer's feed tube. You'll learn from experience what can be added whole and what size chunks work best for your machine. If you have a large feed tube, you won't have to cut up a lot of produce.

- *Some fruits and vegetables don't juice well.* Most produce contains a lot of water, which is ideal for juicing. The vegetables and fruits that contain less water, such as bananas and avocados, will not juice well. They can be used in smoothies and cold soups by first juicing other produce, then pouring the juice into a blender and adding the avocado, for example, to make a raw soup or green smoothie. Mangoes and papayas will juice but make a thicker juice.

- *Drink your juice as soon as you can* after it's made. If you can't drink the juice right away, store it in an insulated container such as a thermos or another airtight, opaque container and in the refrigerator if possible. You can store juice for up to twenty-four hours. Light, heat, and air will destroy nutrients quickly. Be aware that the longer juice sits before you drink it, the more nutrients are lost. You can also freeze the juice.

  If juice turns brown, it has oxidized and lost a large amount of its nutritional value; it is not good to drink it at this point as it may be spoiled. When I was very sick with chronic fatigue syndrome, I had only enough energy to juice once a day. I would store some of the juice for up to twenty-four hours. I got well doing that, so I know the juice had plenty of nutrients even in the stored amount. Melon and cabbage juice do not store well; drink them soon after they've been juiced.

WASTE NOT, WANT NOT

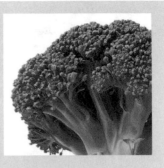

Start saving parts of vegetables to juice that you would normally toss, such as the stems of broccoli, the base of cauliflower, the tough stems of asparagus, radish leaves, kohlrabi leaves, cilantro stems, parsley stems, spinach stems, kale ribs, and any other juicable part I may have overlooked. Add these parts to various juice recipes. If you add them in limited quantity, you won't even know they are there. This is great economy and good for your health. Save your veggie pulp and add it to soups. One of our friends puts veggie pulp in soups and finds it a great addition, as long as she doesn't add too much. Use no more than 2 cups per soup recipe. Save veggie pulp to feed chickens. It gives their eggs bright yellow yokes. You can also compost it for rich garden soil.

And don't forget your pets. I cut off the ends of carrots before juicing, which our Schnauzer, Annie, loves. I also give her some carrot fiber, which she gobbles up.

Look for Organic Produce

The popularity of organic foods has increased dramatically in recent years and continues to grow in popularity. Sales of organic foods reach into the billions of dollars each year and continue to increase annually. It appears that an ever-growing number of people want to avoid the billion pounds or more of pesticides and herbicides sprayed onto or added to crop soil yearly.[3] That's for good reason! It's estimated that only about 2 percent of this amount actually fights insects and weeds while the rest is absorbed into the plants and diffused into our air, soil, and water.[4] This pesticide residue poses long-term health risks, such as cancer, Parkinson's disease, and birth defects,[5] as well as immediate health risks from acute intoxication, including vomiting, diarrhea, blurred vision, tremors, convulsions, and nerve damage.

If pesticides and herbicides do not (as we're told) pose a health risk, then why, when compared with the cancer rates of the general public, is there is a greater incidence of cancer, particularly lymphoma, leukemia, and cancer of the brain, skin, stomach, and prostate among crop workers and farmers and their families?[6]

I'm often asked if organic produce is more nutritious than conventionally grown produce. Studies have shown that it is. According to results from a $25 million study into organic food, the largest of its kind to date, organic produce completely outshines conventional produce in nutritional content. A four-year, European Union–funded study found that organic fruits and vegetables contain up to 40 percent more antioxidants. They have higher levels of beneficial minerals such as iron and zinc. Milk from organic herds contained up to 90 percent more antioxidants. The researchers obtained their results after growing fruits and vegetables and raising cattle on adjacent organic and nonorganic sites. The report also found that eating organic foods can even help to increase the nutrient intake of people who don't eat the recommended number of servings of fruits and vegetables a day.[7]

Additionally, a 2001 study completed as part of a doctoral dissertation at Johns Hopkins University looked at forty-one different studies involving field trials, greenhouse pot experiments, market basket surveys, and surveys of farmers. The most studied nutrients across those surveys included calcium, copper, iron, magnesium, manganese, phosphorus, potassium, sodium, zinc, beta-carotene, and vitamin C. Many studies also looked at nitrates. According to the study there was significantly more vitamin C (27 percent), iron (21 percent), magnesium (29 percent), and phosphorus (13 percent) in the organic produce than in the conventionally grown vegetables. There were also 15 percent fewer nitrates in the organic vegetables. The vegetables that had the biggest increases in nutrients between organic and conventional production were lettuce, spinach, carrots, potatoes, and cabbage.[8] Couple that with the fact that organic produce has less chemical residue, and you can see that buying organically grown food is well worth the effort and the additional cost.

When choosing organically grown foods, look for labels that are marked "certified organic." This means the produce has been cultivated according to strict uniform standards that are verified by independent state or private organizations. Certification includes inspection of farms and processing facilities, detailed record keeping, and pesticide testing of soil and water to ensure that growers and handlers are meeting government standards. You may occasionally see a label that says "transitional organic." This means the produce was grown on a farm that recently converted or is in the process of converting from chemical sprays and fertilizer to organic farming.

You may not be able to afford to purchase everything organic. When that's the case, choose wisely. According to the Environmental Working Group, commercially farmed fruits and vegetables vary in their levels of pesticide residue. Some vegetables, such as broccoli, asparagus, and onions, as well as foods with thicker peels, such as avocados, bananas, and lemons, have relatively low levels of pesticides compared to other fruits and vegetables.[9]

TWO MUST-BUY ORGANIC FOODS

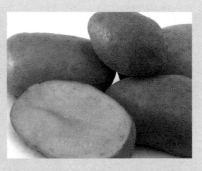

Potatoes are a staple of the American diet. One survey found they account for 30 percent of our overall vegetable consumption. A simple switch to organic potatoes has the potential to have a big impact because commercially farmed potatoes are some of the most pesticide-contaminated vegetables. A 2006 USDA test found that 81 percent of potatoes tested still contained pesticides after being washed and peeled. Also, the potato has one of the highest pesticide contents of forty-three fruits and vegetables tested, according to the Environmental Working Group.[10]

Apples are the second most commonly eaten fresh fruit after bananas, and they are the second most popular fruit juice after orange juice. But apples are also one of the most pesticide-contaminated fruits. The good news is that organic apples are easy to find and readily available in most grocery stores.

Be aware that some vegetables and fruit contain large amounts of pesticide. Each year the Environmental Working Group releases its list of the "Dirty Dozen" fruits and vegetables, which rates fruits and vegetables from worst to best. Eating the least-contaminated vegetables and fruits as found on the "Clean Fifteen" list will expose a person to the least pesticides. You can check it out online at www.ewg.org.

When the organic vegetables or fruit that you want are not available, ask your grocer to get them. You can also look for small-operation farmers in your area and check out farmers markets. Many small farms can't afford to use as many chemicals in farming as large commercial farms use. Another option is to order organic produce by mail, online, or through a co-op.

AVOID THE "DIRTY DOZEN"

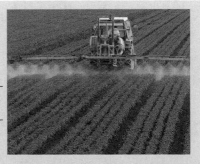

If you can't afford to purchase all organic produce, you can still avoid the worst pesticide-sprayed produce. The nonprofit research organization Environmental Working Group reports periodically on health risks posed by pesticides in produce. This group says you can cut your pesticide exposure by almost 90 percent simply by avoiding the top twelve conventionally grown fruits and vegetables that have been found to be the most contaminated. Studies have shown that eating the twelve most contaminated fruits and vegetables will on average expose a person to about fourteen pesticides per day. Eating the twelve least contaminated vegetables and fruit will expose a person to less than two pesticides per day.[11]

The most current "Dirty Dozen" at the time of this writing is below, ranked in order from the worst to the least contaminated. This year the Environmental Working Group expanded the list to highlight two crops that did not meet the traditional criteria but were commonly contaminated with organophosphate pesticides, highly toxic insecticides that are harmful to the nervous system. Though they have been largely removed from agriculture, these insecticides still show up on some food crops.[12] The "Dirty Dozen" list changes each year, so to get the current ratings, visit www.ewg.org.

1. Apples
2. Celery
3. Sweet bell peppers
4. Peaches
5. Strawberries
6. Nectarines (imported)
7. Grapes (including raisins and wine)
8. Spinach
9. Lettuce
10. Cucumbers
11. Blueberries (domestic)
12. Potatoes

Plus: Green beans and kale/collard greens

Is Irradiated Food Harmful?

Food irradiation exposes food to ionizing radiation in order to destroy microorganisms, bacteria, viruses, or insects that might be present in the food. Stay away from irradiated fruits and vegetables as much as possible. Some food producers use gamma-ray radiation to kill pests, bacteria, and germs in stored food and to increase the food's shelf life. Dr. George Tritsch of Roswell Park Memorial Institute, New York State Department of Health, says he is opposed to consuming irradiated food "because of the abundant and convincing evidence in scientific literature that the condensation products of the free radicals formed during irradiation produce statistically significant increases in carcinogenesis, mutagenesis, and cardiovascular disease in animals and man." There is also reported destruction of vitamins and other nutrients.[13] This practice destroys phytochemicals, biophotons, and enzymes, and it generates harmful by-products such as free radicals (which are toxic and can damage cells) and harmful chemicals known as radiolytic products, which include thalidomide.[14]

Irradiation of fruits and vegetables may pose an even greater problem than irradiation of other foods due to the large quantities

THE ENVIRONMENTAL WORKING GROUP'S "CLEAN FIFTEEN"[15]

These fruits and vegetables are the least contaminated by pesticides.

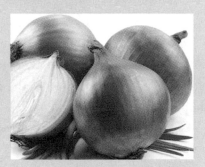

1. Onions
2. Sweet corn
3. Pineapples
4. Avocado
5. Cabbage
6. Sweet peas
7. Asparagus
8. Mangoes
9. Eggplant
10. Kiwi
11. Cantaloupe (domestic)
12. Sweet potatoes
13. Grapefruit
14. Watermelon
15. Mushrooms

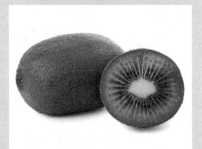

of water found in produce, which allows for greater free-radical production. The answer to food-borne illnesses is not irradiation but stopping the overuse of pesticides, transforming overcrowded factory farm animal lots to humane farms, and ensuring more sanitary conditions in growing produce and food-processing plants.

Stay Away From GMO Foods

Whenever possible, you should avoid genetically modified foods, also known as GMs or GMOs. GMOs (genetically modified organisms) are the result of laboratory techniques by which researchers change plant and farm animal genes to create products with scientifically manufactured proteins or other substances that the human body has no prior experience digesting. Genetically modified plants, for example, may contain non-plant genetic material that may cause the plant to make never-before-encountered chemicals, which the body is unable to process. The altering of plant genes has been done to make plants more resistant to pests, disease, or pesticides; to have a longer shelf life; or to modify ripening.

A recent study carried out by researchers from Monsanto, a leading producer of genetically modified seed, revealed that in experiments on three strains of GM maize (corn), test animals that ate the maize showed signs of liver and kidney damage. Two of the varieties of maize were genetically modified to synthesize toxins used as insecticides, while the third was genetically modified to be resistant to the herbicide Roundup.[16] All three strains of the genetically modified corn are grown and approved for human consumption in America. According to various reports, Monsanto released the raw data only after a legal challenge from Greenpeace and other governmental bodies and groups against genetically modified foods.[17]

The study found that there were unusual concentrations of hormones in the blood and urine of rats fed each strain of the maize for three months when compared with rats given a non-GM diet. Female rats were found to have higher levels of blood sugar and triglycerides. (I pose the question: Could this be one reason many people today have higher levels of blood sugar and triglycerides?) This finding is particularly significant regarding weight loss because it is known that higher blood sugar levels and triglycerides contribute to insulin resistance and metabolic syndrome. The authors of the study concluded, "Effects were mostly associated with the kidney and liver, the dietary detoxifying organs, although different between the 3 GMOs. Other effects were also noticed in the heart, adrenal glands, [and] spleen."[18]

Many genetically modified foods are on grocery store shelves everywhere without protective labeling. We may not know we are buying them. And unsuspecting consumers who may have an allergic reaction to something such as a peanut or Brazil nuts may buy a product with a nut gene that could cause a life-threatening reaction.

We can avoid GMO foods by becoming aware of which foods are most prone to genetic engineering and what products are made from them. Some estimates say that as many as thirty thousand different products on grocery store shelves are "modified." That's largely because many processed foods contain some form of soy. About 90 percent of North America's soy crop is genetically engineered.[19] According to the FDA, more than fifty plant varieties have been examined and approved for human consumption[20]—for example, tomatoes and cantaloupes with modified ripening characteristics; soybeans and sugar beets engineered to be resistant to herbicides; and corn and cotton plants with increased resistance to insect pests.

While all fifty products may not be available in your local supermarket, the prevalence of genetically modified foods in the United States is more widespread than you may think. Deborah Whitman, a senior editor of Cambridge Scientific Abstracts, states, "Highly processed foods, such as vegetable oils or breakfast cereals, most likely contain a small percentage of genetically modified ingredients because the raw ingredients have been pooled into one processing stream from many different sources."[21]

Worldwide, soybeans and corn are the two most widely grown crops, while in the United States soybeans and cotton are the two most prevalent GM crops. The majority of GM crops were modified for herbicide tolerance, with smaller percentages modified for insect pest resistance and for both herbicide tolerance and pest tolerance.

According to Whitman, "Globally, acreage of GM crops has increased twenty-five-fold in just five years, from approximately 4.3 million acres in 1996 to 109 million acres in 2000.... Approximately

99 million acres were devoted to GM crops in the U.S. and Argentina alone."[22]

There are other foods to watch for and buy only organic. Rice is genetically modified to contain high amounts of vitamin A. Sugarcane is genetically modified to be resistant to certain pesticides. A large percentage of sweeteners used in processed food actually come from corn, not sugarcane or beets. Transgenic papayas now cover about three quarters of the total Hawaiian papaya crop. Meat and dairy products often come from animals that have eaten GM feed, which is why it's very important to purchase only pasture-fed, organically raised animal products. Genetically modified peas have created immune responses in mice, suggesting that they could also create serious allergic reactions in people.[23] The peas had been inserted with a gene from kidney beans, which creates a protein that acts as a pesticide. Many vegetable oils and margarines used in restaurants, processed foods, and salad dressings are made from soy, corn, canola, or cottonseed. Unless these oils specifically say "non-GMO" or "organic," they are probably genetically modified.

Even vitamin supplements may be genetically modified: Vitamin C is often made from corn, and vitamin E is usually made from soy. Vitamins A, B_2, B_6, B_{12}, D, and K may have fillers derived from GM corn sources, such as starch, glucose, and maltodextrin.[24] This is precisely the reason we should purchase only high-quality vitamins from reliable sources that use organic materials.

Currently labeling of GMO food is not required; therefore we must become informed consumers and careful shoppers. We can look at the labels of packaged products to see if they contain corn flour or corn-meal, soy flour, cornstarch, textured vegetable protein, corn syrup, or modified food starch. Check the labels of soy sauce, tofu, soy beverages, soy protein isolate, soymilk, soy ice cream, margarine, and soy lecithin, among dozens of other products. If the labels on these foods don't say "organic" or "non-GMO," the chances are strong that they are GMO foods. Check the PLU (price look up) code on the produce stickers at your grocer. Genetically modified food sticker five-digit codes will start with an 8. For example, a genetically modified vine-ripe tomato would be 84805.

As you can see, it's important to make as much of your food from scratch. And when it comes to juicing, it's very important to purchase organically grown and heirloom for produce that is not known to be genetically modified.

CAN GM CORN CAUSE TUMORS?

A two-year French study found that rats fed Monsanto's engineered corn developed large breast tumors, kidney and liver damage, and other serious health problems. The major development of diseases occurred during the thirteenth month of the study. Female rats that ate genetically engineered corn died two to three times more often and more rapidly than rats in the control groups. Meanwhile the males developed tumors that occurred up to a year and a half earlier than rats not fed genetically modified corn.[25]

In addition, results from a ten-year-long study on rats, mice, pigs, and salmon showed that genetically engineered food caused obesity along with significant changes in the animals' digestive systems and major organs, including the liver, kidneys, pancreas, and genitals.[26]

Since the government refuses to mandate the labeling of GMO foods, our only defense is to avoid all corn and soy products (two of the biggest GMO crops in America)—unless the corn or corn product is organic. It's best to avoid all soy no matter what. Even if organic, soy produces many deleterious effects on our health.

Chapter 2

SIMPLE JUICE RECIPES

I F YOU'RE NEW to juicing and want simple, great-tasting recipes to get started, this is the chapter for you. Simple blends such as carrot and apple are a great base to which you can add other ingredients. This is also a great chapter for people in your life who are new to juicing and not quite ready for lots of different combinations.

Do you have picky eaters in your family? Start here or with chapter 5, "Yummy Fruit Juice Blends." For children, simple recipes that incorporate some fruit are probably the best place to start. You can start babies on a single item such as carrot or pear at about six months. Though I don't recommend drinking very much fruit juice, I am also realistic. Young palates and those that have been accustomed to a lot of sweet drinks may never drink juice unless you make it taste really good. That's when adding fruit to juices makes sense. It's still the healthiest thing you or the people you care about could drink. But remember, you can always tuck a few green leaves or a couple sprigs of parsley in a juice, and no one will know it's there.

Apple Cucumber Cooler

½ cucumber
1 green apple
½ lemon, peeled if not organic

Cut produce to fit your juicer's feed tube. Juice ingredients and stir. Pour over ice and drink as soon as possible. Serves 1.

Asparagus Lemonade

2 green apples
6 asparagus stems
½ lemon, peeled if not organic

Cut produce to fit your juicer's feed tube. Juice ingredients and stir. Pour over ice and drink as soon as possible. Serves 1.

Beet-Orange Refresher

2 oranges, peeled
1 small beet with leaves

Cut produce to fit your juicer's feed tube. Juice ingredients and stir. Pour into a glass and drink as soon as possible. Serves 1.

Blueberry-Apple Juice

Studies show that blueberries can help you get rid of belly fat. The effect is thought to be due to the high level of phytochemicals—naturally occurring antioxidants—that blueberries contain. The study also showed that blueberries are helpful in preventing type 2 diabetes. Blueberries can also help fight hardening of the arteries and improve the memory.[1]

1 cup blueberries, fresh or thawed if frozen
2 apples

Cut produce to fit your juicer's feed tube. With the machine off, pour in the berries and top with the plunger to keep the berries from flying out. Then turn the machine on and push the berries through, followed by the apples. Stir the juice and pour into a glass; drink as soon as possible. Serves 1.

Carrot-Cucumber Lemonade

4–5 medium carrots, scrubbed well, tops removed, ends trimmed
1 apple
1 small cucumber, peeled if not organic
1-inch-chunk ginger, peeled
½ medium lemon, peeled if not organic

Cut produce to fit your juicer's feed tube. Juice ingredients and stir. Pour into a glass and drink as soon as possible. Serves 2.

Carrot-Apple Nectar

4-5 carrots, scrubbed well, tops removed, ends trimmed
1 apple

Cut produce to fit your juicer's feed tube. Juice ingredients and stir. Pour into a glass and drink as soon as possible. Serves 1.

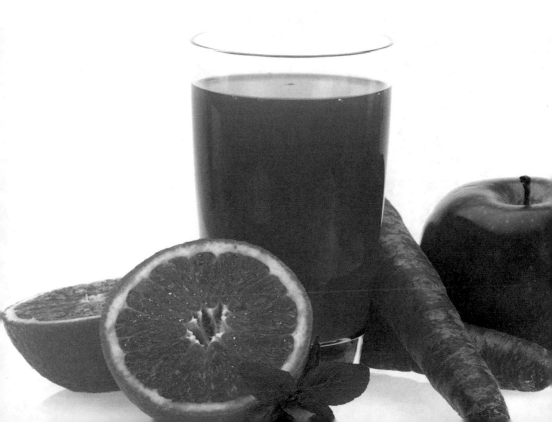

Carrot-Orange-Ginger Cocktail

3–4 carrots, scrubbed well, tops removed, ends trimmed
1 orange, peeled
1-inch-chunk ginger root

Cut produce to fit your juicer's feed tube. Juice ingredients and stir. Pour into a glass and drink as soon as possible. Serves 1.

Cran-Apple Juice

Studies show that cranberries are loaded with acids that researchers believe are useful in dissolving fat deposits. When fat deposits settle in the body, they are hard to get rid of, so it's best to get them before they get "hooked" on you. Some studies suggest that the enzymes in cranberries can aid metabolism, which can also boost weight loss.[2]

1 cup cranberries, fresh or thawed if frozen
2 apples

Cut produce to fit your juicer's feed tube. With the machine off, pour in the berries and top with the plunger, which will keep the berries from flying out. Then turn the machine on and push the berries through, followed by the apples. Stir and pour into a glass. Drink as soon as possible. Serves 1.

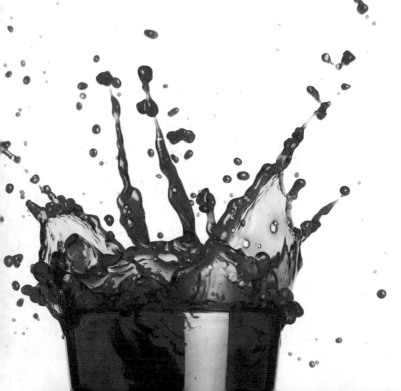

HOW TO AVOID ARSENIC IN APPLE JUICE

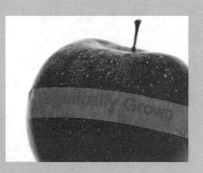

Could your child be consuming harmful levels of arsenic in his or her lunch box apple juice or sippy cup?

You can avoid harmful arsenic by making your own fresh apple juice. When you buy organic apples, you won't be getting the arsenic-laced pesticides. And by juicing your own organic apples, you'll also be getting vitamins, enzymes, and biophotons that are killed in the pasteurization process required for all bottled and packaged juice. You can also make delicious lemonade with two to three apples and one lemon. Add a little spinach or other dark leafy greens, and make beautiful green lemonade.

In 2010 the *St. Petersburg Times* commissioned an independent testing of a number of popular brands of apple juice, including Motts, Apple & Eve Organics, and Walmart's Great Value brand, and found levels of arsenic that have concerned parents and scientists alike.[3] More than a quarter of the eighteen samples tested contained twenty-five to thirty-five parts per billion (ppb) of arsenic. These amounts surpass the FDA's level of concern for heavy metals in juice.

In 2009 a University of Arizona study found similar results, with nine out of ten samples of apple and grape juice containing ten to forty-seven ppb of arsenic.[4] Only one juice—M&B Products of Tampa, which is used for school lunch programs in the region—contained no detectable levels of arsenic in two samples. Dr. Mehmet Oz recently conducted an independent study and also found unsafe levels of arsenic in store-bought apple juice.[5]

Some people have thought there is arsenic in apple seeds, but that is not true. There is a small amount of cyanide, which is found naturally in nature. Arsenic is also found in small amounts in nature and in water—in nature it's an organic version that is not harmful. But the toxic, inorganic version found in store-bought apple juice is harmful and therefore of concern. It is believed that these high arsenic levels are coming from pesticides that contain arsenic.

A large amount of apple juice concentrate that manufacturers are purchasing to make apple juice is coming from China, as well as from Chile, Argentina, and Turkey.[6]

How much arsenic is too much? Richard Wiles, senior vice president for policy at the Environmental Working Group, said, "There's no safe level of arsenic exposure for a kid, and it certainly shouldn't be in these juices."[7] Research has shown a link between lower levels of inorganic arsenic and diabetes, cancer, organ damage, and hormone system disruptions.

To protect you and your family, get out your juicer and make your own apple juice. And you can choose green apples such as pippin or Granny Smith, which have less sugar than other varieties. This also gives you the opportunity to tuck in a few greens that no one in the household might eat, such as parsley, kale, or spinach. Then you can pour a glass or sippy cup of true nutrition that is safe for the whole family to enjoy.

Cucumber Lime Cooler

1 cucumber
1 lime, peeled if not organic

Cut produce to fit your juicer's feed tube. Juice ingredients and stir. Pour over ice in a glass and drink as soon as possible. Serves 1.

Fennel-Apple Juice

¼ fennel bulb with fronds
1–2 green apples

Cut produce to fit your juicer's feed tube. Juice ingredients and stir. Pour into a glass and drink as soon as possible. Serves 1.

Fig-Carrot Cocktail

Researchers have found that a diet rich in raw vegetables and fruit lowers your risk of cancer. Including fresh produce as part of your daily diet has also been associated with fewer deaths from heart attacks and related problems by as much as 24 percent, according to a study published in the *British Medical Journal*.[8]

3–4 carrots, scrubbed well, tops removed, ends trimmed
3–4 fresh figs
½ apple

Cut produce to fit your juicer's feed tube. Juice ingredients and stir. Pour into a glass and drink as soon as possible. Serves 1.

Garlicky Veggie Cocktail

4 carrots, scrubbed well, tops removed, ends trimmed
2-inch-chunk jicama, scrubbed or peeled if not organic
1 lemon, peeled if not organic
1 handful of watercress
1 garlic clove (no need to peel)

Cut produce to fit your juicer's feed tube. Juice ingredients and stir. Pour into a glass and drink as soon as possible. Serves 1–2.

Green Apple-Celery Medley

2 green apples
4 ribs of celery with leaves

Cut produce to fit your juicer's feed tube. Juice ingredients and stir. Pour into a glass and drink as soon as possible. Serves 1.

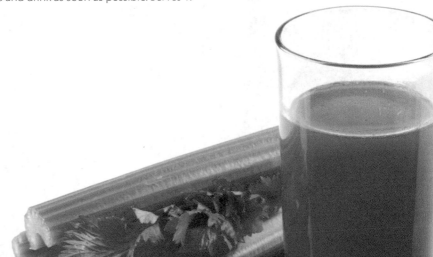

Guava Nectar

2 cups fresh guava, cut into chunks
2 kiwifruit
½ lime, peeled if not organic

Cut produce to fit your juicer's feed tube. Juice ingredients and stir. Pour into a glass and drink as soon as possible. Serves 1.

Happy Beet

2–3 carrots, scrubbed well, tops removed, ends trimmed
1 cucumber, peeled if not organic
1 apple
½ beet with leaves

Cut produce to fit your juicer's feed tube. Juice ingredients and stir. Pour into a glass and drink as soon as possible. Serves 1.

Jicama-Carrot Nectar

2–3 carrots, scrubbed well, tops removed, ends trimmed
1 chunk jicama, approximately 2 inches by 4–5 inches in length with peel, scrubbed

Cut produce to fit your juicer's feed tube. Juice ingredients and stir. Pour into a glass and drink as soon as possible. Serves 1.

Lemonade

2–3 apples
1 lemon, peeled if not organic

Cut produce to fit your juicer's feed tube. Juice ingredients and stir. Pour into a glass and drink as soon as possible. Serves 1.

Lime-Apricot Cooler

1 apple
2 apricots, seeded
½ lime, peeled if not organic

Cut produce to fit your juicer's feed tube. Juice ingredients and stir. Pour into a glass over ice and drink as soon as possible. Serves 1.

Orange-Cucumber Refresher

1 medium to large organic cucumber, peeled if not organic
1 orange, peeled

Cut produce to fit your juicer's feed tube. Juice ingredients and stir. Pour into a glass and drink as soon as possible. Serves 1.

Orange-Radish Refresher

2 oranges, peeled
4 radishes with tops

Cut produce to fit your juicer's feed tube. Juice ingredients and stir. Pour into a glass and drink as soon as possible. Serves 1.

Parsley-Carrot Lemonade

3–4 carrots, scrubbed well, tops removed, ends trimmed
2 apples
1 handful of parsley
1 lemon, peeled if not organic

Cut produce to fit your juicer's feed tube. Juice ingredients and stir. Pour into a glass and drink as soon as possible. Serves 1.

Pepper Upper

3–4 carrots, scrubbed well, tops removed, ends trimmed
½ cucumber, peeled if not organic
¼ bell pepper (green, red, or yellow)

Cut produce to fit your juicer's feed tube. Juice ingredients and stir. Pour into a glass and drink as soon as possible. Serves 1.

Pineapple-Asparagus Cocktail

6 asparagus stems
1 lime, peeled if not organic
¼ pineapple, peeled if not organic

Cut produce to fit your juicer's feed tube. Juice ingredients and stir. Pour into a glass and drink as soon as possible. Serves 1.

Red Sunrise

1 green apple
½ small beet with leaves
1 cucumber, peeled if not organic

Cut produce to fit your juicer's feed tube. Juice ingredients and stir. Pour into a glass and drink as soon as possible. Serves 1.

Simply Tomato

2 medium vine-ripened tomatoes
4 radishes with tops, washed
1 lime or lemon, peeled if not organic

Cut produce to fit your juicer's feed tube. Juice ingredients and stir. Pour into a glass and drink as soon as possible. Serves 1.

Spicy Orange

1 orange, peeled
1 cucumber, peeled if not organic
1-inch-chunk ginger root

Cut produce to fit your juicer's feed tube. Juice ingredients and stir. Pour into a glass and drink as soon as possible. Serves 1.

Sweet Tomato

3–4 carrots, scrubbed well, tops removed, ends trimmed
1 green apple
1 tomato

Cut produce to fit your juicer's feed tube. Juice ingredients and stir. Pour into a glass and drink as soon as possible. Serves 1.

Tomato-Celery Blend

2 tomatoes
2 ribs of celery with leaves

Cut produce to fit your juicer's feed tube. Juice ingredients and stir. Pour into a glass and drink as soon as possible. Serves 1.

Waldorf Morning

1 green apple
3 ribs of celery with leaves
1 lemon, peeled if not organic
½ cucumber, peeled if not organic

Cut produce to fit your juicer's feed tube. Juice ingredients and stir. Pour into a glass and drink as soon as possible. Serves 1.

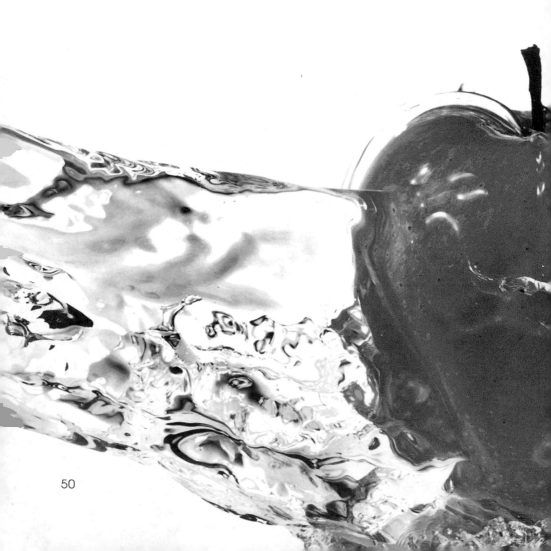

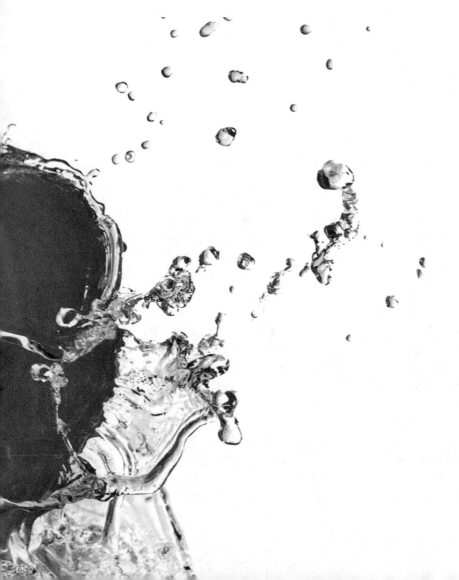

Chapter 3

GOURMET AND EXOTIC JUICE BLENDS

WHEN YOU'RE READY to venture into more interesting juice blends or would like to try more flavors and unique juice combinations, this is the chapter for you. It's always a good idea to choose a wide variety of whole foods in your diet so that you get a wide complement of nutrients. I had so much fun developing these recipes and giving them entertaining names. They are different from the norm and really delicious. I hope you enjoy them too.

I also hope the variety in these juice recipes will inspire you to stick with the juicing lifestyle program. Then you too may experience wonderful changes in your body, just as Lisa did.

> My whole life I've tried to find ways to eat better and improve my health. I followed my mom's determination not to believe the medical doctors who told her that her health problems were in her head. The fatigue that she felt did not exist, they told her, and she needed a psychiatrist.
>
> My health journey began at age thirteen when I gave up pasteurized milk. Around age eighteen I cut out red meat, and at twenty-two I eliminated sodas. Instead of going to doctors when I got sick, I would try vitamins, herbs, and other supplements. I did get results and was able to stay pretty healthy over the years. But I knew the foods in my diet weren't everything my body needed.
>
> I always had little symptoms that bothered me. I started getting spider veins in my legs and ridges in my fingernails. Occasionally I would lose hair for a couple of

months. I just couldn't get rid of a few extra pounds. It was hard for me to wake up in the morning. And alternative health professionals would tell me that my digestion wasn't good and that my liver was congested. They gave me supplements to take. But it just didn't seem right to keep taking supplements to fix these things, especially when they weren't getting fixed.

I believed vegetables were at least part of the solution, so I spent many years trying to prepare them in ways that I could live with. The best I could do was put them in a blender and will myself to drink them. That only worked part of the time. The rest of the time they went to waste.

In July 2011 I watched a YouTube video of Cherie talking with Dr. Mercola about juicing. I bought her book and read about the health challenges she has had in her life. I had heard about juicing before, but I didn't try it because I had heard the juicer was expensive and hard to clean. Also it just didn't seem right to throw away so much of the vegetable pulp. But after hearing Cherie's story, I was determined to try it.

I decided to buy a juicer and a fridge full of vegetables. I started an eight-day juice fast the same day someone close to me was having surgery to remove a cancerous tumor. I drank only juice for those first eight days. I lost eight pounds! That's one pound a day! The weight loss was encouraging, but I didn't really feel any better or have any symptoms disappear during this time.

This diet change was hard for me at first. For the first week I struggled with which vegetables to buy, the preparation and cleanup time, and not really feeling any better. I kept referring back to Cherie's book to follow the recipes and eventually became more comfortable with which vegetables to use. I found helpful tips in her book to cut down on preparation time.

It took about two months before I started to see improvements in other areas. But then my digestion improved. My circulation has also improved. And I keep seeing other signs of improvement all the time. Even my fingernails are growing straighter and stronger. I'm now happy to have vegetables by juicing as part of my life and not by forcing or gagging them down as I had been when they were blended.

Cherie's passion about juicing got my attention. Because of her, I have found juicing is easier than I thought it would be. And I'm more satisfied than I thought I'd be. Cherie's program is making juicing easy to stick with.

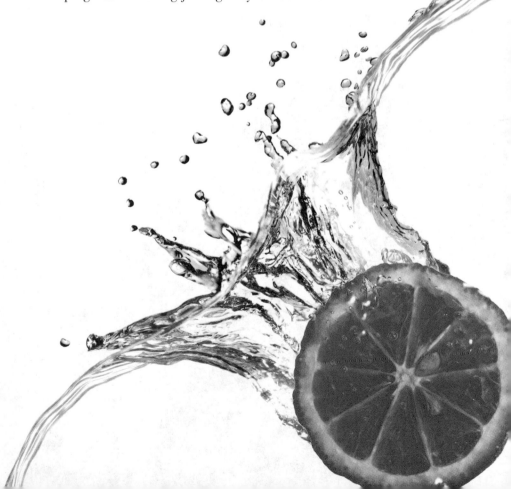

Asian Delight

2-inch by 4- to 5-inch chunk of jicama, scrubbed well or peeled
2–3 carrots, scrubbed well, tops removed, ends trimmed
1 daikon radish, trimmed and scrubbed
1-inch-chunk ginger root

Cut produce to fit your juicer's feed tube. Juice ingredients and stir. Pour into a glass and drink as soon as possible. Serves 1.

Asian Pear Juice With Beet and Baby Greens

1 Asian pear
1 handful of baby greens
1 small beet with leaves and stems

Cut produce to fit your juicer's feed tube. Juice ingredients and stir. Pour into a glass and drink as soon as possible. Serves 1.

Basil-Nectarine Lemonade

2 nectarines, pits removed
1 green apple
1 small handful of fresh basil
1 lemon, peeled if not organic

Cut produce to fit your juicer's feed tube. Juice ingredients and stir. Pour into a glass and drink as soon as possible. Serves 1.

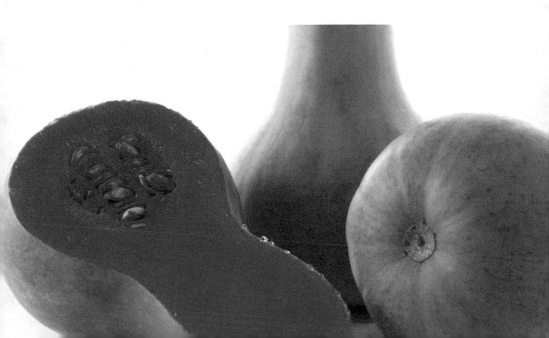

Blushing Carrot

6 carrots, scrubbed well, tops removed, ends trimmed
8 strawberries, with caps
1-inch-chunk ginger root

Cut produce to fit your juicer's feed tube. Juice ingredients and stir. Pour into a glass and drink as soon as possible. Serves 1.

Brussels Delight

1 large vine-ripened tomato
2 romaine lettuce leaves
8 organic string beans
3 brussels sprouts
1 lemon, peeled if not organic

Cut produce to fit your juicer's feed tube. Juice ingredients and stir. Pour into a glass and drink as soon as possible. Serves 1.

Butternut Squash and Apple Juice

4–5 strips of butternut squash, cut in strips ½ inch by 4 inches
1 apple
1–2 kale leaves
2 ribs of celery with leaves
1-inch-chunk ginger root

Cut produce to fit your juicer's feed tube. Juice ingredients and stir. Pour into a glass and drink as soon as possible. Serves 1.

Cabbage Patch

4 carrots, scrubbed well, tops removed, ends trimmed
1 small lemon, peeled if not organic
1 green apple
1 small wedge red or green cabbage
1-inch-chunk ginger root

Cut produce to fit your juicer's feed tube. Juice ingredients and stir. Pour into a glass and drink as soon as possible. Serves 1–2.

Caliente Fiesta

1 cucumber, peeled if not organic
2-inch by 4- to 5-inch chunk of jicama, scrubbed well or peeled
¼ small jalapeño pepper, seeds removed unless you like really hot foods

Cut produce to fit your juicer's feed tube. Juice ingredients and stir. Pour into a glass and drink as soon as possible. Serves 1.

Chili Lime

4- to 5-inch by 2- to 3-inch chunk jicama, scrubbed or peeled if not organic
1 lime, peeled if not organic
¼ small jalapeño pepper, seeds removed unless you like really hot foods

Cut produce to fit your juicer's feed tube. Juice ingredients and stir. Pour into a glass and drink as soon as possible. Serves 1.

Cucumber Dill

1 cucumber, peeled if not organic
1 lime, peeled if not organic
2 sprigs fresh dill

Cut produce to fit your juicer's feed tube. Juice ingredients and stir. Pour into a glass and drink as soon as possible. Serves 1.

Fennel-Carrot-Orange Cocktail

3–4 carrots, scrubbed well, tops removed, ends trimmed
1 fennel bulb with fronds
1 orange, peeled

Cut produce to fit your juicer's feed tube. Juice all ingredients. Pour into a glass and drink as soon as possible. Serves 2.

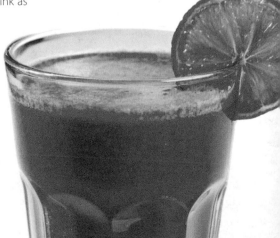

THERMOGENIC FOODS REV UP YOUR METABOLISM

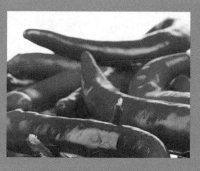

Thermogenesis means the production of heat, which raises metabolism and burns calories. Thermogenic foods are essentially fat-burning foods and spices that help increase your metabolism. This means that with some of your kitchen staples, you can burn fat during or right after you eat and increase your fat-burning potential just by eating them. So include these superfoods often in your juices.

Hot peppers. One study found that the animals studied developed obesity mainly because they didn't produce enough heat after eating, not because the animals ate more or were less active.[1] A recent study found that hot peppers turn up the internal heat, which helps in burning calories.[2] You can add hot peppers or a dash of hot sauce to many juice recipes, and they'll taste delicious.

Garlic. When it comes to weight loss, garlic appears to be a miracle food. A team of doctors at Israel's Tel Hashomer Hospital conducted a test on rats to find out how garlic can prevent diabetes and heart attacks, and they found an interesting side effect—none of the rats given allicin (a compound in garlic) gained weight.[3] Garlic is a known appetite suppressant. The strong odor of garlic stimulates the satiety center in the brain, thereby reducing feelings of hunger. It also increases the brain's sensitivity to leptin, a hormone produced by fat cells that regulates appetite. Further, garlic stimulates the nervous system to release hormones such as adrenaline, which speed up metabolic rate. This means a greater ability to burn calories. More calories burned means less weight gained—a terrific correlation.

Ginger. Ginger contains a substance that stimulates gastric enzymes, which can boost metabolism. The better your metabolism, the more calories you will burn. Ginger has been shown to be an anti-inflammatory—inflammation is implicated in obesity and heart disease. It helps improve gastric motility—the spontaneous peristaltic movements of the stomach that aid in moving food through the digestive system. When the digestive system is functioning at its best, you'll experience less bloating and constipation.

It has also been found to lower cholesterol. And ginger is the top vegan source of zinc, which gives a big boost to your immune system. Top that off with the fact that it tastes delicious in juice recipes, and you have a super spice. I add it to almost every juice recipe I make.

Fennel-Watercress-Cucumber

1 handful of watercress
1 dark green lettuce leaf
1 cucumber, peeled if not organic
½ fennel bulb and fonds
1 lemon, peeled if not organic

Cut produce to fit your juicer's feed tube. Wrap watercress in lettuce leaf and push through juicer slowly. Juice all remaining ingredients. Pour into a glass, stir, and drink as soon as possible. Serves 1.

Four-Veggie Supreme

2 tomatoes
½ fennel bulb with fronds
2 ribs of celery with leaves
1 handful of flat-leaf parsley
½ tsp. Celtic sea salt

Cut produce to fit your juicer's feed tube. Juice produce ingredients and stir. Pour into a glass, stir in sea salt, and drink as soon as possible. Serves 2.

Fresh Fennel-Pear

2 fennel bulbs with fronds
2 ribs of celery with leaves
1 pear

Cut produce to fit your juicer's feed tube. Juice all ingredients. Pour into a glass and drink as soon as possible. Serves 1.

Fresh Garden Medley

¼ small head red cabbage
4 ribs of organic celery with leaves
4 carrots, scrubbed well, tops removed, and ends trimmed
1 dark green lettuce leaf
½-inch-chunk ginger root

Cut produce to fit your juicer's feed tube. Juice ingredients and stir. Pour into a glass and drink as soon as possible. Serves 1–2.

Garlic Delight

1 handful of parsley
1 dark green lettuce leaf
½ medium cucumber, peeled if not organic
1 garlic clove
3 carrots, scrubbed well, tops removed, ends trimmed
2 ribs of celery with leaves

Wrap the parsley in the lettuce leaf. Juice the cucumber then the parsley-lettuce wrap. Push the garlic through the juicer with the carrots. Follow with the celery. Stir and pour into a glass. Drink as soon as possible. Serves 1–2.

Ginger Twister

1 handful of parsley
1 kale leaf
1 apple
½ lemon, peeled if not organic
3 carrots, scrubbed well, tops removed,
    ends trimmed
2-inch-chunk fresh ginger root

Cut produce to fit your juicer's feed tube. Wrap parsley in kale leaf and push slowly through juicer. Follow with remaining ingredients and stir. Pour into a glass and drink as soon as possible. Serves 1.

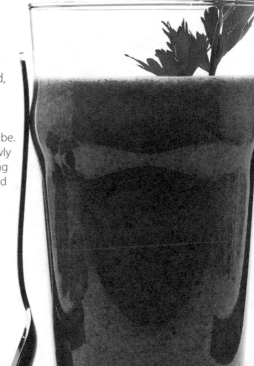

Golden Cress

1 small handful of watercress
1 dark green lettuce leaf
5 carrots, scrubbed well, tops removed, ends trimmed
1 apple

Cut produce to fit your juicer's feed tube. Wrap watercress in lettuce leaf and push through juicer slowly. Juice all remaining ingredients. Pour into a glass, stir, and drink as soon as possible. Serves 2.

Gourmet Live

1 small handful of parsley
1 cup loosely packed baby spinach leaves
3 dark green lettuce leaves
4 carrots, scrubbed well, tops removed, ends trimmed
½ green pepper, including seeds and inner membrane
2 green onions
1 garlic clove (you don't need to peel)
2 ribs of celery with leaves
½ small beet with leaves

Cut produce to fit your juicer's feed tube. Wrap parsley and spinach in lettuce leaves and push through the juicer. Follow with the remaining ingredients. Pour into glasses and drink as soon as possible. Serves 2.

Granny's Special

3–4 carrots, scrubbed well, tops removed, ends trimmed
2 Granny Smith apples
2 ribs of celery with leaves
1 pear
1-inch-chunk ginger root

Cut produce to fit your juicer's feed tube. Juice all ingredients. Pour into a glass and drink as soon as possible. Serves 2.

Grapefruit, Fennel, and Spring Greens

½ fennel bulb with fronds
1 handful of spring greens
1 red grapefruit, peeled

Cut produce to fit your juicer's feed tube. Juice ingredients and stir. Pour into a glass and drink as soon as possible. Serves 1.

Happy Mary

1 large cucumber, peeled if not organic
1 tomato
3 ribs of celery with leaves
1 lemon, peeled if not organic
⅛ tsp. hot sauce
Pinch Celtic sea salt
Pinch black pepper

Cut produce to fit your juicer's feed tube. Juice cucumber, tomato, celery, and lemon. Stir in hot sauce, sea salt, and pepper. Serve chilled over ice. Serves 2.

Happy Sombrero

4–5 carrots, scrubbed well, tops removed, ends trimmed
1 lime, peeled if not organic
1-inch-chunk fresh ginger root
Pinch of cayenne pepper

Cut produce to fit your juicer's feed tube. Juice ingredients and stir in cayenne pepper. Pour into a glass and drink as soon as possible. Serves 1.

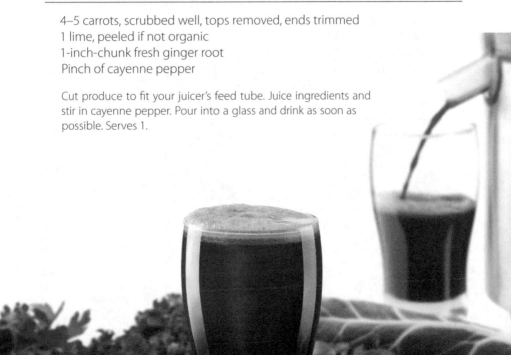

JUICING HELPS IMPROVE BRAIN HEALTH

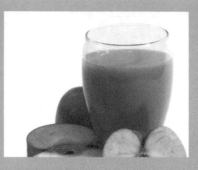

The brain is one of the organs that are particularly sensitive to free-radical damage and oxidative stress. It is very important to include lots of antioxidants in your diet to protect your brain. Juicing is one of the best ways you can accomplish that. There are a number of studies showing that juice helps to improve brain function. According to one study published in the Journal of Alzheimer's Disease, a growing body of evidence demonstrates that we can take steps to delay age-related cognitive decline, including Alzheimer's disease. A team of researchers at Neurodegeneration Research University of Massachusetts found that drinking apple juice helped mice perform better than normal in maze trials and prevented the decline in performance observed in aged mice. The researchers observed that mice drinking the human equivalent of two glasses of apple juice per day for one month produced less of a small protein fragment called "beta-amyloid," which is responsible for forming senile plaques that are commonly found in the brains of individuals suffering from Alzheimer's disease. The researchers concluded that regular consumption of apple juice can help to keep one's mind functioning at its best and may delay Alzheimer's disease.[4]

Hot Tomato

2 medium tomatoes
1 small handful of parsley
2 dark green lettuce leaves
2 radishes with leaves
1 lime or lemon, peeled if not organic
Dash of hot sauce

Cut produce to fit your juicer's feed tube. Wrap parsley in lettuce leaves and push through juicer slowly. Juice all remaining ingredients and stir in hot sauce. Pour into a glass and drink as soon as possible. Serves 1.

Lemon-Fennel on Ice

1 fennel bulb with fronds
1 cucumber, peeled if not organic
1 lemon, peeled if not organic

Cut produce to fit your juicer's feed tube. Juice all ingredients and pour over ice. Serves 2.

Lime Cordial

2 green apples
1 lime, peeled if not organic
1–2 drops stevia
1 cup sparkling water

Juice the apples and lime. Pour into a glass, and add the stevia and sparkling water. Add ice. Stir and drink as soon as possible. Serves 1.

Mango-Cucumber Salsa Cooler

1 firm, ripe mango, peeled and seeded
1 cucumber, peeled if not organic
1 handful of cilantro
1 small lime, peeled if not organic
½ orange, peeled

Cut produce to fit your juicer's feed tube. Juice all ingredients and stir. Pour into a glass and drink as soon as possible. Serves 2.

Mint Julep

2 bunches of fresh mint
1 dark green lettuce leaf
2 apples

Cut produce to fit your juicer's feed tube. Wrap mint in lettuce leaf and push through juicer slowly, followed by apples. Pour into a glass over ice, stir, and drink as soon as possible. Serves 1.

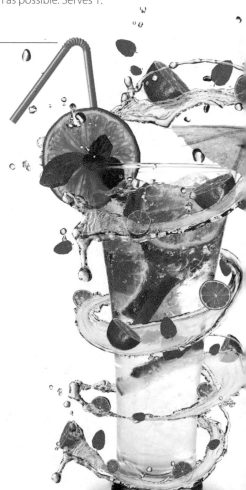

Moroccan Tomato

1 handful of parsley
1 green lettuce leaf
2 tomatoes
1 small handful of cilantro
1-inch-chunk ginger root
½ cucumber, peeled if not organic
⅛ tsp. cumin
Dash of paprika
Dash of cinnamon

Cut produce to fit your juicer's feed tube. Wrap parsley in lettuce leaf and push through juicer slowly. Juice the tomatoes, cilantro, ginger root, and cucumber. Stir in the herbs and spices. Pour into glasses and drink as soon as possible. Serves 2.

My Garden Delight

1 handful of parsley
1 kale leaf
3 carrots, scrubbed well, tops removed, ends trimmed
2 ribs of celery with leaves
1 collard leaf
1 tomato
1 broccoli stem

Cut produce to fit your juicer's feed tube. Wrap parsley in kale leaf and push through juicer slowly. Juice remaining ingredients and stir. Pour into glasses and drink as soon as possible. Serves 2.

Nectarine Salsa Cocktail

3 ripe large nectarines, pits removed
1 lime, peeled if not organic
1 handful of cilantro
½ cucumber, peeled if not organic
¼ small fresh serrano or jalapeño pepper, seeds removed unless you like really hot foods

Cut produce to fit your juicer's feed tube. Juice ingredients and stir. Pour into a glass and drink as soon as possible. Serves 1.

Orange-Mint Julep

2 oranges, peeled
1 lemon, peeled if not organic
1 bunch mint

Cut produce to fit your juicer's feed tube. Juice ingredients and stir. Pour into a glass over ice and drink as soon as possible. Serves 1.

Papaya Bliss

1 ripe medium papaya with seeds, peeled
2–3 carrots, scrubbed well, tops removed, ends trimmed
1 lemon, peeled if not organic
1-inch-chunk ginger root

Cut produce to fit your juicer's feed tube. Juice ingredients and stir. Pour into a glass over ice and drink as soon as possible. Serves 1.

Parsnip-Carrot-Orange

2–3 carrots, scrubbed well, tops removed, ends trimmed
1 parsnip
1 orange, peeled if not organic

Cut produce to fit your juicer's feed tube. Juice ingredients and stir. Pour into a glass and drink as soon as possible. Serves 1.

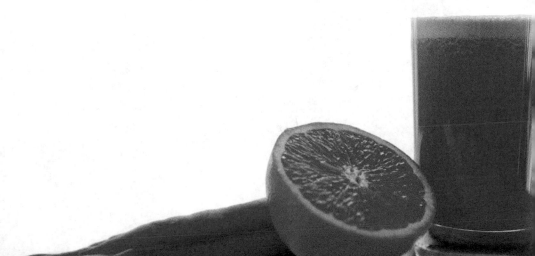

Peppy Piña Colada

1 lime, peeled if not organic
4 kale, chard, or collard leaves
¼ pineapple, peeled if not organic
½ cup coconut water

Juice the lime, greens, and pineapple. Pour into a glass; add the coconut water and ice. Stir and drink as soon as possible. Serves 2.

Perky Parsley

1 bunch of parsley
2 dark green lettuce leaves
3 carrots, scrubbed well, tops removed, ends trimmed
2 ribs of celery with leaves
1 cucumber, peeled if not organic
1 lemon, peeled if not organic

Cut produce to fit your juicer's feed tube. Wrap parsley in lettuce leaves and push through juicer slowly. Juice remaining ingredients and stir. Pour into a glass and drink as soon as possible. Serves 1–2.

Pineapple Kicker

¼ pineapple, peeled if not organic
6 kale leaves
2 ribs of celery with leaves
1-inch-chunk ginger root

Cut produce to fit your juicer's feed tube. Juice ingredients and stir. Pour into a glass and drink as soon as possible. Serves 1.

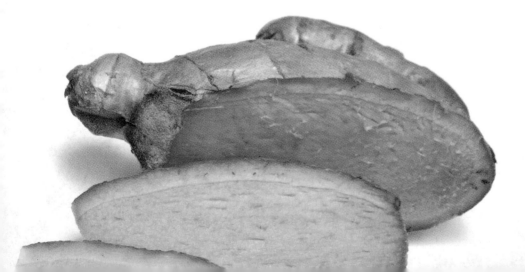

Pippin Party

1 small handful of parsley
1 green lettuce leaf
3–4 carrots, scrubbed well, tops removed, ends trimmed
2 ribs of celery with leaves
2 cloves of garlic
2 pippin apples

Cut produce to fit your juicer's feed tube. Warp parsley in lettuce leaf and push through juicer slowly. Juice all remaining ingredients and stir. Pour into a glass and drink as soon as possible. Serves 1.

Pumpkin Patch

1 cup cubed pumpkin, skin removed (you can juice the seeds)*
1–2 apples
½ cucumber, peeled if not organic
2 ribs of celery with leaves

Cut produce to fit your juicer's feed tube. Juice ingredients and stir. Pour into a glass and drink as soon as possible. Serves 1.

*Note: Pumpkin is very hard and can be a challenge for smaller juicers, but not for heavy-duty machines. Be sure to cut the pumpkin into pieces small enough for your juicer.

Quince and Spice

1 large quince
1 apple
1 lemon, peeled if not organic
Dash of cinnamon
Dash of nutmeg

Cut produce to fit your juicer's feed tube. Juice ingredients and stir in cinnamon and nutmeg. Pour into a glass and drink as soon as possible. Serves 1.

Radish-Kohlrabi Delight

5 carrots, scrubbed well, tops removed, ends trimmed
5–6 radishes with leaves
1 cucumber, peeled if not organic, or 1 large chunk of jicama
1 lemon, peeled if not organic
½ kohlrabi* with leaves

Cut produce to fit your juicer's feed tube. Juice all the ingredients. Stir the juice and pour into a glass. Serve at room temperature or chilled, as desired. Serves 1.

*Note: Use the other half of the kohlrabi, sliced thinly, in a salad.

Rawsome Veggies

1 cup spinach, packed
2 kale leaves
1 tomato
3 ribs of celery with leaves
4 carrots, scrubbed well, tops removed, ends trimmed
½ small beet with leaves
1 green onion
1 lime, peeled if not organic

Cut produce to fit your juicer's feed tube. Wrap spinach in kale leaves and push through juicer slowly. Juice all remaining ingredients and stir. Pour into glasses and drink as soon as possible. Serves 2.

Red Cabbage-Jicama-Carrot-Lime Juice

1 handful of flat-leaf parsley leaves
1 green lettuce leaf
3–4 carrots, scrubbed well, tops removed, ends trimmed
2-inch by 4- to 5-inch chunk of jicama, scrubbed well or peeled
¼ small red cabbage
1 lime, peeled if not organic

Cut produce to fit your juicer's feed tube. Wrap parsley in lettuce leaf and push through juicer slowly. Juice remaining ingredients and stir. Pour into a glass and drink as soon as possible. Serves 1.

Red Sunset

1 blood orange, peeled
4 purple kale leaves
¼ red cabbage
1 lemon, peeled if not organic
½ small beet with leaves
¼ bunch mint
1-inch-chunk ginger root

Cut produce to fit your juicer's feed tube. Juice ingredients and stir. Pour into a glass and drink as soon as possible. Serves 2.

Refreshing Mint Cooler

1 fennel bulb and fronds
1 cucumber, peeled if not organic
1 green apple such as Granny Smith or pippin
1 handful of mint

Cut produce to fit your juicer's feed tube. Juice ingredients and stir. Pour into a glass over ice and drink as soon as possible. Serves 1–2.

Revitalizing Tomato-Coconut Juice

Coconut water is rich in electrolytes, which revitalize the body.

1 cup carrot juice (about 6 medium carrots)
Juice of 1 lemon
1 tomato, cut into chunks and frozen
1 large handful of cilantro
½ cup coconut water

Pour carrot and lemon juice into a blender. Add the frozen tomato chunks and cilantro. Blend until the tomato chunks are completely processed. Stir in the coconut water. Pour into glasses and be revitalized. Serves 2.

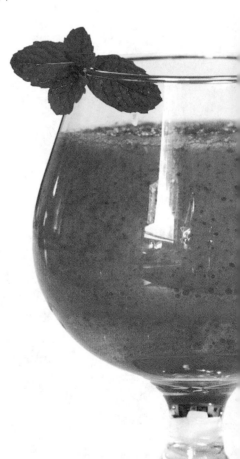

Rockin' Tomato

1 cup loosely packed flat-leaf parsley
1 dark green lettuce leaf
2 tomatoes
1 fennel bulb and fronds
2 ribs of celery with leaves
1 green onion
Pinch of Celtic sea salt

Cut produce to fit your juicer's feed tube. Wrap parsley in lettuce leaf and push through juicer. Juice remaining ingredients, add sea salt, and stir. Pour into a glass and drink as soon as possible. Serves 2.

Santa Fe Salsa Cocktail

1 medium tomato
1 cucumber, peeled if not organic
1 small handful of cilantro
1 lime, peeled if not organic
Dash of hot sauce (optional) or ¼ jalapeño pepper, seeds removed unless
    you like really hot foods

Cut produce to fit your juicer's feed tube. Juice ingredients, add hot sauce, and stir. Pour into a glass and drink as soon as possible. Serves 1.

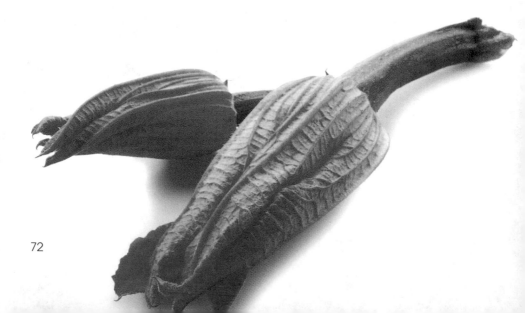

Siesta Refresher

4 sprigs of parsley
2 dark green lettuce leaves
2 medium vine-ripened tomatoes
2 radishes with leaves
1 lime, peeled if not organic

Cut produce to fit your juicer's feed tube. Wrap parsley in lettuce and push through juicer slowly. Juice remaining ingredients and stir. Pour into a glass and drink as soon as possible. Serves 1.

Southwest Spicy Tomato

1 small handful of cilantro
1 small handful of parsley
2 dark green lettuce leaves
2 medium tomatoes
1 lime, peeled if not organic
½ jalapeño pepper, seeds removed unless you like really hot foods

Cut produce to fit your juicer's feed tube. Wrap cilantro and parsley in lettuce leaves and push through the juicer slowly. Juice all remaining ingredients and stir. Pour into two glasses and drink as soon as possible. Serves 2.

Spring Honeydew

½ honeydew melon with seeds and rind if organic
1 small handful of basil
1 small handful of fresh mint
1 lime, peeled if not organic

Cut produce to fit your juicer's feed tube. Juice ingredients and stir. Pour in a glass and drink as soon as possible. Serves 2.

Squash Blossom Surprise

3–4 squash blossoms
1 large heirloom tomato
4 sprigs fresh basil
2 ribs of celery with leaves

Cut produce to fit your juicer's feed tube. Juice ingredients and stir. Pour into a glass and drink as soon as possible. Serves 1.

Sweet Chili-Lime

2 oranges, peeled
1 lime, peeled if not organic
½ small jalapeño pepper, seeds removed unless you like really hot foods

Cut produce to fit your juicer's feed tube. Juice all ingredients and drink as soon as possible. Serves 1.

Sweet Rhubarb

3 carrots, scrubbed well, tops removed, ends trimmed
2 stalks rhubarb (no leaves; they are toxic)
2 leaves romaine lettuce
1 apple
1 lemon, peeled if not organic
1-inch-chunk ginger root

Cut produce to fit your juicer's feed tube. Juice ingredients and stir. Pour into a glass and drink as soon as possible. Serves 1–2.

Tangy Tomato

½ cup flat-leaf parsley
1 green lettuce leaf
3 medium tomatoes
1–2 tomatillos, with skin
4 carrots, scrubbed well, tops removed, ends trimmed
½ cup flat-leaf parsley
1 garlic clove
1 lemon, peeled if not organic
½ tsp. tamari or low-sodium soy sauce

Cut produce to fit your juicer's feed tube. Wrap parsley in lettuce leaf and push through juicer. Juice remaining ingredients and stir in tamari or soy sauce. Pour into a glass and drink as soon as possible. Serves 2.

Thai Cabbage Cocktail

4 carrots, scrubbed well, tops removed, ends trimmed
½ lemon, peeled if not organic
¼ small head green cabbage
4 sprigs fresh mint
1–2 drops stevia, optional
Dash coriander
Pinch Celtic sea salt

Cut produce to fit your juicer's feed tube. Juice ingredients and stir in stevia as desired, coriander, and sea salt. Pour into a glass and drink as soon as possible. Serves 1.

The Big Apple

2 apples
1 handful of spinach
1 lemon, peeled if not organic
1-inch-chunk ginger root

Cut produce to fit your juicer's feed tube. Juice ingredients and stir. Pour into a glass and drink as soon as possible. Serves 1.

Tomatillo Kicker

5 fresh tomatillos with skins
3 radishes with leaves
1 cucumber, peeled if not organic
1 handful of cilantro
1 lemon, peeled if not organic

Cut produce to fit your juicer's feed tube. Juice ingredients and stir. Pour into a glass and drink as soon as possible. Serves 1–2.

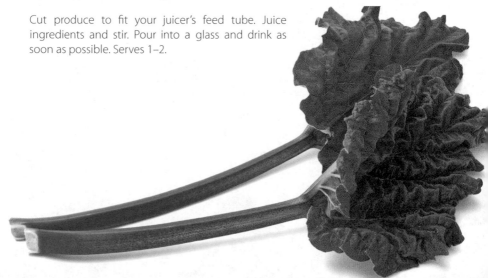

Tomato Florentine With a Twist

2 vine-ripened tomatoes
4–5 sprigs basil
1 large handful of spinach
1 lemon or lime, peeled if not organic

Juice one tomato. Wrap the basil in several spinach leaves. Turn off the machine and add the spinach and basil. Turn the machine back on and gently tap to juice them. Juice the remaining tomato and lemon. Stir juice, pour into a glass, and drink as soon as possible. Serves 1.

Turnip and Fennel

½ turnip with leaves
4 carrots, scrubbed well, tops removed, ends trimmed
1 apple
¼ fennel bulb and fronds
2 ribs of celery with leaves

Cut produce to fit your juicer's feed tube. Juice ingredients and stir. Pour into a glass and drink as soon as possible. Serves 1.

Veggie Delight

1 cucumber, peeled if not organic
2–3 ribs of celery with leaves
½ organic lemon with peel
1-inch-chunk ginger root

Cut produce to fit your juicer's feed tube. Juice ingredients and stir. Pour into a glass and drink as soon as possible. Serves 1–2.

Virgin Mary

2 tomatoes
2 ribs of celery with leaves
1 lemon, peeled if not organic
Dash of hot sauce
Dash of black pepper
Dash of Celtic sea salt

Cut produce to fit your juicer's feed tube. Juice tomatoes, celery, and lemon; stir in hot sauce, pepper, and salt. Pour into a glass over ice, and drink as soon as possible. Serves 1.

Watermelon-Cucumber-Jicama Cocktail

1 large chunk of watermelon, about ⅛ of a small melon, with rind if organic
1 cucumber, peeled if not organic
¼ jicama, scrubbed, or peeled if not organic

Cut produce to fit your juicer's feed tube. Juice ingredients and stir. Pour into a glass and drink as soon as possible. Serves 2.

Watermelon-Ginger-Yellow Tomato

1 large chunk of watermelon, about ⅛ of a small melon, with rind if organic
1 yellow tomato
1-inch-chunk ginger root

Cut produce to fit your juicer's feed tube. Juice ingredients and stir. Pour into a glass and drink as soon as possible. Serves 2.

Watermelon–Red Pepper Salsa Cocktail

1 large chunk of watermelon, about ⅛ of a small melon, with rind if organic
¼ cantaloupe with seeds, with rind
    if organic
½ red bell pepper with seeds and
    membranes
1 small lime, peeled if not organic
1 small handful of cilantro
¼ small jalapeño pepper, seeds
    removed unless you like really
    hot foods
4 fresh mint sprigs

Cut produce to fit your juicer's feed tube. Juice ingredients and stir. Pour into a glass and drink as soon as possible. Serves 2.

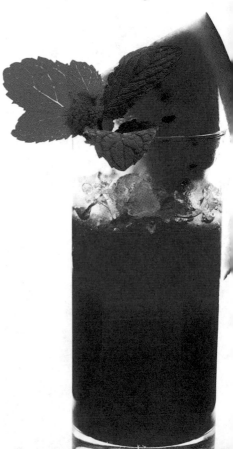

Winter Squash-Orange-Celery

¼ winter squash, cut into thin strips (otherwise it's very hard to juice)
1 orange, peeled
2 ribs of celery with leaves
½ cucumber, peeled if not organic

Cut produce to fit your juicer's feed tube. Juice ingredients and stir. Pour into a glass and drink as soon as possible. Serves 1.

Yucatecan Orange

2 oranges, peeled
3 kale leaves
1 garlic clove (no need to peel)
Pinch of Celtic sea salt
Pinch of black pepper
Pinch of allspice

Cut produce to fit your juicer's feed tube. Juice oranges, kale, and garlic; stir in spices. Pour into a glass and drink as soon as possible. Serves 1.

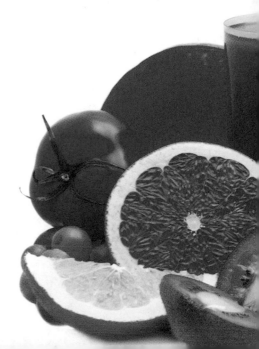

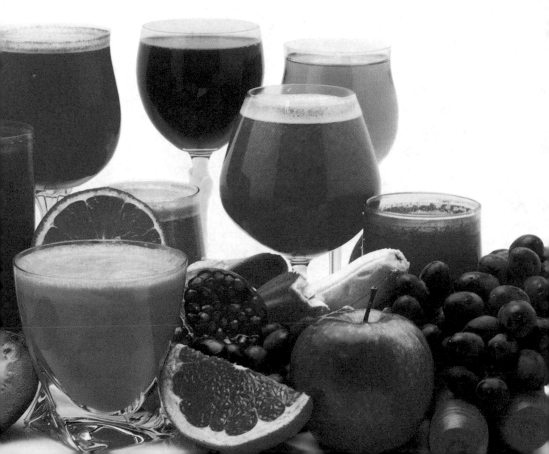

Chapter 4

GREEN JUICE RECIPES

IT IS BELIEVED that our ancient ancestors ate up to six pounds of green leaves per day when the plants were in season. We can envision them walking from one place to another, picking leaves as they went. Can you imagine eating a grocery bag full of greens every day during the right seasons? Few of us eat even the minimum USDA recommendation of five servings of vegetables and fruit a day or three cups of dark green vegetables per week. And yet these veggies deliver a bonanza of vitamins, minerals, enzymes, biophotons, and phytonutrients. The good news is that you can juice them and easily consume one to three cups of greens per day.

Calorie for calorie, dark green leafy vegetables are among the most concentrated sources of nutrition. They are a rich source of minerals, including iron, calcium, potassium, and magnesium—plus vitamins K, C, E, and many of the B vitamins. They also provide a variety of phytonutrients, including alpha- and beta-carotene, lutein, and zea-xanthin, which protect our cells from damage and our eyes from age-related diseases. Dark green leaves even contain small amounts of omega-3 fats.

Juicing is one way you can get these power-packed beautifiers into your diet every day. There are many greens that can be juiced, such as collard leaves, chard, beet tops, kale, kohlrabi leaves, mustard greens, parsley, spinach, lettuce, cilantro, watercress, arugula, and dandelion greens. All you need is a juicer and some great-tasting recipes to make a significant change in your health. I'm excited to share Brenda's story with you. Juicing changed her health and her life.

You are a huge inspiration and invaluable resource, Cherie, and I thank you! I found your work after a difficult second pregnancy and even worse recovery. After dealing with ITP (idiopathic thrombocytopenic purpura), I developed hyperthyroidism/post-partum thyroiditis, which eventually turned into hypothyroidism. I also had my gallbladder removed with complications. It's now seven weeks since having my second baby via C-section. Juicing has been a huge life-changer on the road to recovery. It even helped with some of the baby fat weight loss. So again, thank you for putting all of this out there.

I read that kale and beets were good for raising platelets. Some people with low platelets can increase the iron in their diet with these foods, and that raises the platelet count. I have noticed that I stopped craving chocolate and soda since I've been juicing. I finally feel satisfied. Now, if I'm not juicing diligently and have a craving, I look up in your book why I'm craving something and eat what I need. It's very interesting! My doctors have been pleased with my results, and all of them have strongly encouraged me to continue juicing. I look forward to your future work. You're making a huge difference!

Alkaline Power

3 carrots, scrubbed well, tops removed, ends trimmed
2 ribs of celery with leaves
1 handful of spinach
1 cucumber, peeled if not organic
½ green apple

Cut produce to fit your juicer's feed tube. Juice all ingredients and stir. Pour into a glass and drink as soon as possible. Serves 1.

Amazing Green Drink

1 small kohlrabi with leaves
1 kale leaf
1 kiwifruit
1 rib of celery with leaves
1 apple (green has less sugar)
½ lemon, peeled if not organic

Cut produce to fit your juicer's feed tube. Roll the leaves and push through the juicer with the kiwifruit and celery rib. Follow with the apple and lemon. Stir and drink as soon as possible. Serves 1.

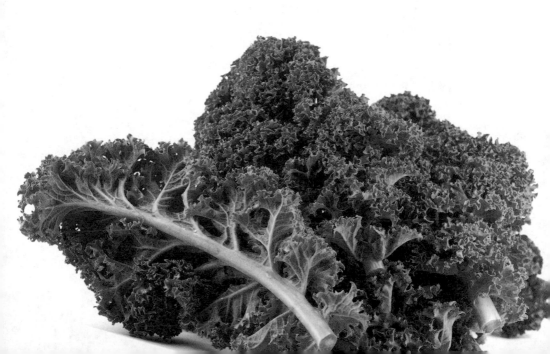

Apple-Cucumber Lite

2 apples
2 ribs of celery with leaves
1 cucumber, peeled if not organic
1-inch-chunk ginger root

Cut produce to fit your juicer's feed tube. Juice all ingredients and stir. Pour into a glass and drink as soon as possible. Serves 1.

Arugula-Apple-Lemon

1 cucumber, peeled if not organic
1 lemon, peeled if not organic
1 green apple
1 small handful of arugula

Cut produce to fit your juicer's feed tube and push through the juicer. Stir and serve as soon as possible. Serves 1.

Beet Express

3 carrots, scrubbed well, tops removed, ends trimmed
2 kale leaves
1 small beet with green leaves
1-inch-chunk ginger root
1 lemon, peeled if not organic
1 clove garlic

Cut produce to fit your juicer's feed tube. Juice all ingredients, stir, and drink as soon as possible. Serves 1.

Broccoli Surprise

Broccoli could help reverse the damage diabetes inflicts on blood vessels. The key is likely a compound in the vegetable called sulforaphane, which encourages production of enzymes that protect the blood vessels and reduces the number of molecules that cause cell damage, known as reactive oxygen species (ROS), by up to 73 percent.

1–2 carrots, scrubbed well, tops removed, ends trimmed
2–3 broccoli florets or 1 broccoli stem[*]
2 ribs of celery with leaves
1 cucumber, peeled if not organic
1 lemon, peeled if not organic

Cut produce to fit your juicer's feed tube. Juice all ingredients, stir, and drink as soon as possible. Serves 1.

* Note: Save all broccoli stems and juice them; you can add them to most recipes and reap the rewards. This is good economy and adds great nutrition.

JUICE RECIPES FOR DIABETICS AND PREDIABETICS

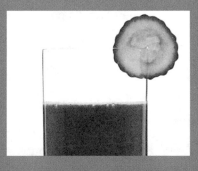

Often people will tell me they can't juice because they have diabetes. If you have diabetes or other sugar metabolism problems, you can juice vegetables, but you should choose low-sugar veggies and only low-sugar fruit such as lemon, lime, and cranberries. Carrots and beets would be too high in sugar by themselves, but you could add a small amount of either of them to a green juice recipe and dilute them with cucumber, which has plenty of water. Most other fruit are higher in sugar and should be avoided. Berries are low in sugar, especially cranberries, and can be added to juice recipes. Green apples are lower in sugar than yellow or red but should still be used very sparingly.

If you have diabetes, this of all the chapters in this book is your juice chapter. But even here, not all recipes are recommended for you. So choose the recipes that only use the fruits lemon, lime, cranberries, or rhubarb, and plenty of greens. Dark leafy greens are an excellent source of magnesium, and there is a connection between low magnesium intake and diabetes. I've worked with people who have reversed diabetes by juicing low-sugar vegetables and eating many more living foods along with a low-glycemic diet.

Captain Kidd's Green Drink

3 green leaves such as kale, chard, collards, or dark green lettuce
2 oranges, peeled
1 cup strawberries with caps

Cut produce to fit your juicer's feed tube. Juice all ingredients, stir, and serve as soon as possible. Serves 1.

Chard Lemonade

2 green apples
1 lemon, peeled if not organic
5 leaves of chard

Cut produce to fit your juicer's feed tube and push through the juicer. Stir and serve as soon as possible. Serves 1.

Cherie's Morning Blend

Rather than coffee, why not wake up your body with an energizing, delicious juice?

4–5 carrots, scrubbed well, tops removed, ends trimmed
4 dark green leaves, such as chard, kale, or collards
2 ribs of celery with leaves
1 large cucumber, peeled if not organic
1 lemon peeled, if not organic
1-inch-chunk ginger root

Cut produce to fit your juicer's feed tube. Juice ingredients and stir. Pour into a glass and drink as soon as possible. Serves 2.

Cilantro-Mint-Jalapeño

1 cucumber, peeled if not organic
1 bunch of spearmint
1 bunch of cilantro
1 lime, peeled if not organic
¼ jalapeño pepper, seeds removed unless you like really hot foods

Cut produce to fit your juicer's feed tube. Juice all ingredients, stir, and drink as soon as possible. Serves 1.

Cool Cucumber

1 cucumber, peeled if not organic
2 ribs of celery with leaves
2 leaves baby bok choy
2 romaine lettuce leaves
2–3 carrots, scrubbed well, tops removed,
    ends trimmed
3–4 sprigs cilantro
3–4 sprigs mint
1 lime, peeled if not organic

Cut produce to fit your juicer's feed tube. Juice all ingredients, stir, and drink as soon as possible. Serves 2.

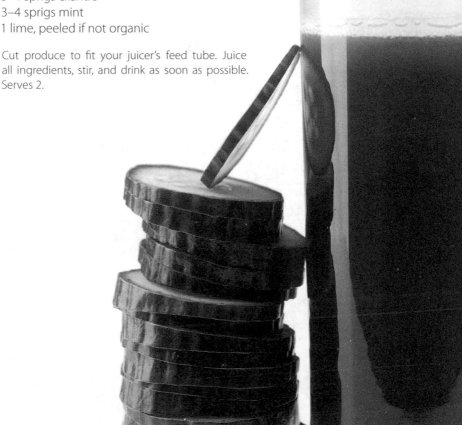

Cucumber-Tomato-Cilantro Cooler

2 tomatoes
1 handful of cilantro
1 cucumber, peeled if not organic
1 lime, peeled if not organic

Cut produce to fit your juicer's feed tube. Juice all ingredients. Pour over ice, stir, and serve chilled. Serves 2.

Dandelion-Coconut Water

Dandelion greens are quite bitter. You can add a sweet fruit such as an apple if you like.

1 bunch dandelion greens
1 lime, peeled if not organic
1 cup coconut water

Juice the dandelion greens and lime; stir in coconut water, and serve immediately. Serves 1.

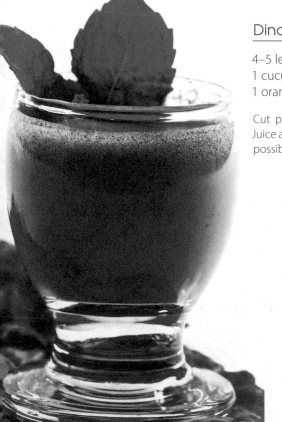

Dino Delight

4–5 leaves dino kale
1 cucumber, peeled if not organic
1 orange, peeled

Cut produce to fit your juicer's feed tube. Juice all ingredients, stir, and drink as soon as possible. Serves 1.

Field of Greens

3 romaine lettuce leaves
2 ribs of celery with leaves
2 kale leaves
1 green apple or 1 pear
1 lemon, peeled if not organic

Cut produce to fit your juicer's feed tube. Juice all ingredients, stir, and drink as soon as possible. Serves 1.

Fitness Combo

1 handful of parsley
1 handful of spinach
2 lettuce leaves
3–4 carrots, scrubbed well, tops removed, ends trimmed
1 small beet with greens
1 rib of celery with leaves
¼ green pepper
2 cloves garlic (you don't need to peel)
1-inch-chunk ginger root

Wrap parsley and spinach in lettuce leaves. Cut all ingredients to fit your juicer's feed tube. Push lettuce wraps through the juicer, followed by the remaining ingredients. Stir and serve as soon as possible. Serves 2.

Garden Patch

1 handful of flat-leaf parsley
1 handful of spinach
3 leaves romaine lettuce
4 carrots, scrubbed well, tops removed, ends trimmed
2 ribs of celery with leaves

Wrap parsley and spinach in lettuce leaves. Cut remaining ingredients to fit your juicer's feed tube. Push lettuce wraps through the juicer with carrots and celery. Stir and serve as soon as possible. Serves 2.

Goin' Green

4 beet leaves
4 kohlrabi leaves
2 ribs of celery with leaves
1 cucumber, peeled if not organic
2–3 carrots, scrubbed well, tops removed, ends trimmed
1 pear
½ lemon, peeled if not organic

Place some of the green leaves in your juicer; alternate remaining leaves with celery followed by cucumber, carrot, pear, and lemon. Stir the juice and drink as soon as possible. Serves 1–2.

Green Bean Pro

Green beans are good for the pancreas and help stabilize blood sugar levels.

2–3 carrots, scrubbed well, tops removed, ends trimmed
1 handful of fresh green beans
2 ribs of celery with leaves
1 cucumber, peeled if not organic
1 lemon, peeled if not organic

Cut produce to fit your juicer's feed tube. Juice all ingredients, stir, and drink as soon as possible. Serves 1.

Green Cocktail

1 handful of parsley
2 chard leaves
2 collard leaves
1 cucumber, peeled if not organic
1 lemon, peeled if not organic

Wrap parsley inside a chard or collard leaf, and then push all leaves through the juicer with the cucumber. Follow with the lemon. Stir the juice and drink as soon as possible. Serves 1–2.

SPRINKLE CINNAMON ON YOUR JUICE

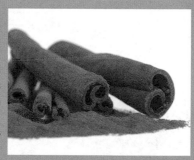

Researchers have suggested that people with diabetes or hypoglycemia may see improvements by adding ¼ to 1 teaspoon of cinnamon to their food. A twelve-week London study involved fifty-eight type 2 diabetics. After twelve weeks on about ½ teaspoon of cinnamon per day, study subjects had significantly lower blood sugar levels and significantly reduced blood pressure.[1]

Green Delight

1 handful of parsley
1 handful of spinach
2 chard leaves
1 rib of celery with leaves
1 apple (green is lower in sugar)
½ lemon, peeled if not organic

Cut produce to fit your juicer's feed tube. Wrap the parsley and spinach in the chard leaves and push through the juicer with the celery. Juice the apple and lemon. Stir the juice and drink as soon as possible. Serves 1.

Green Goodness

6 sprigs parsley
3 leaves dino kale
2 ribs of celery with leaves
1 cucumber, peeled if not organic
1 fennel stalk and fronds

Cut produce to fit your juicer's feed tube. Wrap parsley in kale leaves and push through juicer slowly. Juice remaining ingredients and stir. Pour into a glass and drink as soon as possible. Serves 1.

Green Supreme

1 handful of parsley
1 small handful of cilantro
1 chard leaf
2 ribs of celery with leaves
1 cucumber, peeled if not organic
1 green apple
1 lemon, peeled if not organic
1-inch-chunk ginger root

Cut produce to fit your juicer's feed tube. Wrap parsley and cilantro in the chard leaf. Start with celery and cucumber, and then push the chard-parsley-cilantro wrap through the juicer slowly; follow with remaining ingredients. Pour into a glass and drink as soon as possible. Serves 2.

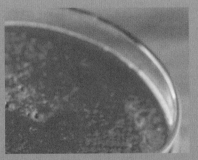

GREEN JUICE ON A MISSION

Even if you took the time to chew up a couple of cups of green veggies each day, you wouldn't get as much benefit from them as you will from juicing them. The mechanical process of juicing the vegetables makes the difference because it breaks apart the plant-cell walls and allows your body to absorb it better than even the best-chewed food. Juicing has an effect like throwing marbles instead of tennis balls at a chain-link fence—juiced contents are going to go through your intestinal tract in a way that "tennis-ball-size" nutrients can't.

Juice contains easily absorbed micronutrients that will optimize your overall health and wellness. Green juices energize your body, fire up your metabolism, speed weight loss, and reboot your health.

Greens for Life

4 ribs of celery with leaves
4 kale leaves
1 green apple
1 cucumber, peeled if not organic
1-inch-chunk ginger root
1 lemon, peeled if not organic

Cut produce to fit your juicer's feed tube. Juice ingredients and stir. Pour into a glass and drink as soon as possible. Serves 1.

La Bella With Greens

In Italian this means "a beautiful life with greens."

1 apple (green is lower in sugar)
1 lemon, peeled if not organic
½ red pepper with seeds
3 ribs of celery with leaves
1 cucumber, peeled if not organic
4 romaine lettuce leaves

Cut produce to fit your juicer's feed tube. Start with the apple and lemon, and juice all ingredients and stir. Pour into a glass and drink as soon as possible. Serves 2.

Lean Mean Green Juice

1 handful of spinach
1 handful of parsley
2 kale leaves
2 ribs of celery with leaves
1 cucumber, peeled if not organic
1-inch-chunk ginger root
½ pear
½ green apple

Cut produce to fit your juicer's feed tube. Wrap spinach and parsley in kale leaves. Start with celery and cucumber; then push the kale wraps through slowly. Follow with remaining ingredients. Pour into a glass and drink as soon as possible. Serves 2.

Lettuce Wrap

1 handful of spinach
1 small handful of parsley
2 green lettuce leaves
3 ribs of celery with leaves
2 asparagus stems
1 large tomato

Cut produce to fit your juicer's feed tube. Wrap spinach and parsley in lettuce leaves. Start with celery, then juice lettuce wraps, followed by asparagus and tomato. Stir and pour into a glass; drink as soon as possible. Serves 1–2.

GREENS, MAGNESIUM, HEALTH, AND WEIGHT LOSS

Juice your greens—they're rich in magnesium, known as nature's Valium! Magnesium is critical for more than three hundred chemical reactions in your body, and unfortunately most Americans are deficient in this mineral. In fact, it may be the single most important nutritional deficiency in the United States.

Many studies have shown that even a small amount of magnesium has a major effect on preventing heart attacks. Magnesium also has been called the "antistress mineral." It plays a vital role in fighting off stress, relaxes muscles, prevents osteoporosis, builds healthy bones, supports restful sleep, prevents restless leg syndrome, prevents constipation, boosts energy, calms the body, and relieves tension.

Magnesium also helps us lose weight. A lack of magnesium is a definite contributor to weight gain and obesity. When magnesium is low, cells don't recognize insulin and glucose accumulates in the blood—then it gets stored as fat instead of being burned for fuel. Further, magnesium helps prevent fat storage.

When magnesium levels drop too low, it can trigger hyperventilation and panic attacks, even seizures, if severe. Such symptoms can be relieved by increasing dietary magnesium. In addition to juicing greens, if you take magnesium supplements, use only absorbable forms such as magnesium citrate or glycinate.

Magnesium-rich greens include:

- Chard
- Collards
- Beet tops
- Parsley
- Spinach
- Kohlrabi leaves
- Kale
- Dandelion greens
- Lettuce (dark green)
- Mustard greens

Magnesium Special

4–5 beet tops
2 Swiss chard leaves
2 collard leaves
1 cucumber, peeled if not organic
½ green apple (omit if diabetic)
½ lemon, peeled if not organic

Cut produce to fit your juicer's feed tube. Juice ingredients and stir. Pour into a glass and drink as soon as possible. Serves 2.

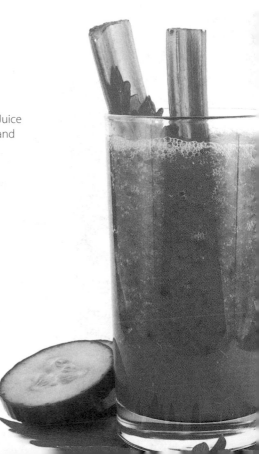

Mint at the Market

1 bunch of fresh mint
5 kale leaves
2 ripe pears

Cut produce to fit your juicer's feed tube. Wrap mint in a kale leaf. Start with half of the pear, then push the kale wrap through the juicer slowly; follow with remaining ingredients. Pour into a glass and drink as soon as possible. Serves 1.

Mint-Chard Lemonade

1 small handful of mint
3 chard leaves
2 apples
1 lemon, peeled if not organic

Cut produce to fit your juicer's feed tube. Wrap the mint in a chard leaf and push through your juicer. Follow with the remaining ingredients. Pour into a glass and drink as soon as possible. Serves 1–2.

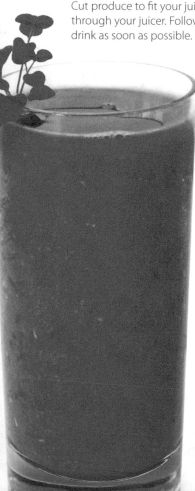

Misty Garden

1 small handful of parsley
2–3 kale leaves
3 carrots, scrubbed well, tops removed, ends trimmed
1 apple
1-inch-chunk ginger root

Cut produce to fit your juicer's feed tube. Wrap parsley in a kale leaf. Juice the carrots first, then push the kale wrap through slowly; follow with remaining ingredients. Pour into a glass and drink as soon as possible. Serves 1.

Moroccan Beet

1 small bunch of mint
1 lettuce leaf
1 beet, with leaves
1 cucumber, peeled if not organic
1 lemon, peeled if not organic

Cut produce to fit your juicer's feed tube. Wrap mint in lettuce leaf. Start by juicing the beet and cucumber, then push the lettuce-mint wrap through slowly, and follow with lemon. Pour into a glass and drink as soon as possible. Serves 1.

Multi-Sprout Drink

1 cucumber, peeled if not organic
2 ribs of celery with leaves
1 small handful of sprouts such as broccoli or radish
1 large handful of sunflower sprouts
1 small handful of buckwheat sprouts
1 lemon, peeled if not organic

Cut produce to fit your juicer's feed tube. Juice ingredients and stir. Pour into a glass and drink as soon as possible. Serves 1.

Papaya-Spinach Cooler

1 papaya, with seeds, peeled
1 cup loosely packed baby spinach
1 lime, peeled if not organic
½ cup coconut water

Juice the papaya, spinach, and lime. Pour the juice in a glass over ice and add the coconut water. Stir and drink as soon as possible. Serves 1.

Parsley-Fennel-Celery Delight

1 handful of parsley
1 green lettuce leaf
2 ribs of celery with leaves
1 cucumber, peeled if not organic
1 lime, peeled if not organic

Cut produce to fit your juicer's feed tube. Wrap parsley in lettuce leaf. Start by juicing the celery and cucumber, then push the lettuce-parsley wrap through the juicer slowly, and follow with the lime. Pour into a glass, stir, and drink as soon as possible. Serves 2.

Pineapple-Spinach-Mint

¼ pineapple, peeled if not organic
1 handful of spinach

4 sprigs of mint Cut produce to fit your juicer's feed tube. Start with half of the pineapple followed by spinach, mint, and then the remaining pineapple. Stir the juice and pour into a glass. Drink as soon as possible. Serves 1.

MAGNESIUM SUPPLEMENTS OR GREEN JUICE?

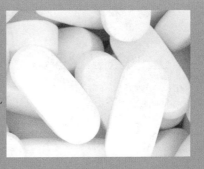

The particles in magnesium supplements are too large for the body to completely absorb, which makes the magnesium in green juice far superior. Green plants take inorganic minerals from the soil through their tiny roots and incorporate them into their cells, turning them into very absorbable organic minerals. These mineral particles are much smaller and easier for the body to absorb than those found in supplements. It is estimated that more than 90 percent of a plant's minerals is delivered to the cells when you juice greens. So juice up those beautiful leaves! And here's the good news—you'll increase your energy exponentially. That means you'll get more done and feel more like working out, so you'll burn more calories and build more muscle.

Red Sails in the Sunset

3 carrots, scrubbed well, tops removed, ends trimmed
½ red bell pepper with seeds and membrane
1 small beet with leaves
1 leaf red Swiss chard
1 lemon, peeled if not organic

Cut produce to fit your juicer's feed tube. Juice all ingredients and stir. Pour into a glass and drink as soon as possible. Serves 1.

Red-Green Cocktail

3 carrots, scrubbed well, tops removed, ends trimmed
3 leaves red Swiss chard
1 green apple
1 wedge red cabbage
1 lime, peeled if not organic

Cut produce to fit your juicer's feed tube. Juice all ingredients. Stir and pour into a glass. Drink as soon as possible. Serves 1.

Rio Fiesta

1 orange, peeled
4 romaine lettuce leaves
½ small jicama, peeled if not organic
4 red radishes with leaves

Cut produce to fit your juicer's feed tube. Start with the orange and juice all ingredients and stir. Pour into a glass and drink as soon as possible. Serves 1.

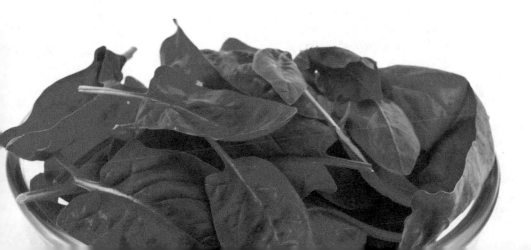

Simply Green

1 handful of spinach
1 handful of parsley
4 kale leaves
1 cucumber, peeled if not organic
3 ribs of celery with leaves
1 clove garlic (no need to peel)

Cut produce to fit your juicer's feed tube. Wrap spinach and parsley in the kale leaves. Start with half the cucumber; then push the kale wraps through the juicer slowly. Follow with remaining ingredients and stir. Pour into a glass and drink as soon as possible. Serves 1.

Spicy Spinach-Grapefruit

1 cup fresh, loosely packed baby spinach
1 lettuce leaf
¼ medium jicama, peeled if not organic
½ red grapefruit, peeled
1-inch-chunk ginger root

Cut produce to fit your juicer's feed tube. Wrap spinach in the lettuce leaf. Start with jicama; then push the lettuce wrap through juicer slowly. Follow with remaining ingredients and stir. Pour into a glass and drink as soon as possible. Serves 1.

Spinach Power Up

½ cucumber, peeled if not organic
1 small handful of parsley
1 green lettuce leaf
3 carrots, scrubbed well, tops removed, ends trimmed
2 ribs of celery with leaves
½ beet, scrubbed well, with stem and leaves
½ lemon, peeled if not organic

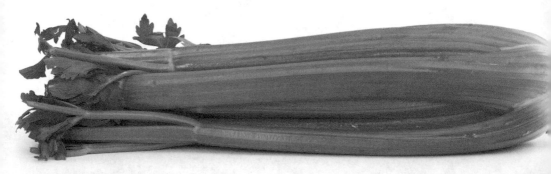

Cut produce to fit your juicer's feed tube. Start with cucumber; then wrap parsley in lettuce leaf and push through the machine slowly. Juice all remaining ingredients and stir. Pour into a glass and drink as soon as possible. Serves 1–2.

Spinach-Peach Delight

2 peaches, seeded
2 handfuls of spinach

Cut produce to fit your juicer's feed tube. Juice ingredients and stir. Pour into a glass and drink as soon as possible. Serves 1.

Spring Greens-Fennel-Sprout Cocktail

3 fennel stalks and fronds
1 handful of wild chicory leaves
1 handful of mixed spring greens
½ cup broccoli sprouts
3 ribs of celery with leaves

Cut produce to fit your juicer's feed tube. Juice ingredients and stir. Pour into a glass and drink as soon as possible. Serves 1.

Sprout-Cucumber Recharger

1 cucumber, peeled if not organic
1 handful of sunflower sprouts (optional)
1 handful of buckwheat sprouts (optional)
1 small handful of clover sprouts (optional)
2 kale leaves
1 large handful of spinach
1 lime, peeled if not organic

Cut the cucumber to fit your juicer's feed tube. Juice half of the cucumber first. Bunch up the sprouts (if using) and wrap in one kale leaf, then wrap the spinach in the other kale leaf. Turn off the machine and add them to the juicer. Turn the machine back on and push the kale leaves through slowly with the rest of the cucumber, then juice the remaining cucumber and lime. Stir ingredients, pour into a glass, and drink as soon as possible. Serves 1–2.

Summer Love

4 ribs of celery with leaves
1 handful of parsley
4 chard leaves
4 apricots, seeds removed
2 peaches, seeds removed

Cut produce to fit your juicer's feed tube. Start with the celery. Wrap parsley in a chard leaf and push through the juicer slowly. Juice remaining ingredients and stir. Pour into a glass and drink as soon as possible. Serves 1.

Super Green

1 pear
1 lemon, peeled if not organic
4 kale leaves
2 ribs of celery with leaves
1 cucumber, peeled if not organic
1-inch-chunk ginger root

Cut produce to fit your juicer's feed tube. Start with the pear and lemon, and juice all ingredients and stir. Pour into a glass and drink as soon as possible. Serves 2.

Super Sprout Drink

1 small handful of clover or radish sprouts
1 large handful of sunflower sprouts
1 small handful of buckwheat sprouts
2 kale leaves
1 cucumber, peeled if not organic

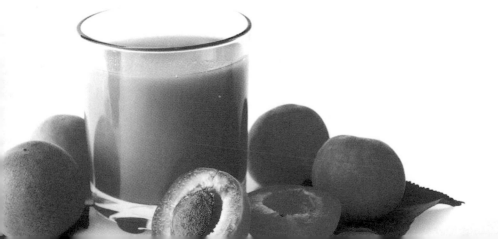

Cut produce to fit your juicer's feed tube. Wrap sprouts in kale leaves and push through juicer slowly. Juice remaining ingredients and stir. Pour into a glass and drink as soon as possible. Serves 1.

Sweet Alkaline Rejuvenator

3 kale leaves
1 chunk of watermelon (approximately 2 inch by 4 inch) with rind, if organic
1 lime, peeled if not organic
½ beet with leaves

Cut all ingredients to fit your juicer's feed tube. Juice all ingredients, stir, and drink as soon as possible. Serves 1.

Sweet Green Sombrero

1 red or yellow apple
3 carrots, scrubbed well, tops removed, ends trimmed
2 ribs of celery with leaves
2 kale leaves
1 cucumber, peeled if not organic
1 lemon, peeled if not organic
¼ jalapeño pepper, seeds removed unless you like really hot foods

Cut produce to fit your juicer's feed tube. Start with apple and juice all ingredients. Stir, pour into a glass, and drink as soon as possible. Serves 2.

Sweet Serenity

1 handful of spinach
1 romaine leaf
1 apple
2 ribs of celery with leaves
1 cucumber, peeled if not organic
1 lime, peeled if not organic

Cut produce to fit your juicer's feed tube. Wrap spinach in the romaine leaf. Start with apple; then push the lettuce wrap through juicer slowly. Follow with remaining ingredients and stir. Pour into a glass and drink as soon as possible. Serves 1.

Tomatillo Salsa Cocktail

5–6 fresh tomatillos
1 handful of cilantro
1 lime, peeled if not organic
1 garlic clove (no need to peel)
¼ small jalapeño pepper, seeds removed unless you like really hot foods

Cut produce to fit your juicer's feed tube. Juice all ingredients and stir. Pour into a glass and drink as soon as possible. Serves 1.

Tomato-Cucumber-Dill Drink

2 tomatoes
1 cucumber, peeled if not organic
1 stalk fresh dill weed

Cut produce to fit your juicer's feed tube. Juice all ingredients and stir. Pour into a glass and drink as soon as possible. Serves 1.

Tom-Tom

3 carrots, scrubbed well, tops removed, ends trimmed
1 handful of spinach
1 dark green lettuce leaf
1 tomato
1 tomatillo
1 lime, peeled if not organic

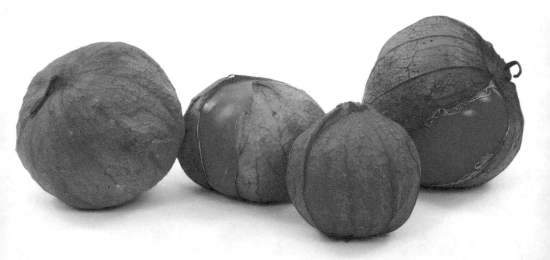

Cut produce to fit your juicer's feed tube. Start by juicing the carrots. Wrap the spinach in the lettuce leaf and push through the juicer. Follow with remaining ingredients and stir. Pour into a glass and drink as soon as possible. Serves 2.

Totally Green

1 handful of parsley
1 handful of spinach
5 green lettuce leaves
2 ribs of celery with leaves
2 green apples (yellow or red for a sweeter taste)

Cut produce to fit your juicer's feed tube. Wrap the parsley and spinach in the lettuce leaves and push through the juicer slowly with the celery and apple. Stir the juice and drink as soon as possible. Serves 1.

V-8 Charger

1 tomato
1 handful of spinach
1 small handful of parsley
1 kale leaf
2 lettuce leaves
3 carrots, scrubbed well, tops removed, ends trimmed
2 ribs of celery with leaves
1 lemon, peeled if not organic

Cut produce to fit your juicer's feed tube. Start by juicing tomato. Wrap spinach and parsley in kale and lettuce leaves and push through juicer slowly. Then juice all remaining ingredients and stir. Pour into glasses and drink as soon as possible. Serves 2.

Veggie Tales

4–5 carrots, scrubbed well, tops removed, ends trimmed
3 ribs of celery with leaves
1 broccoli stem
1 cucumber, peeled if not organic
1 kale leaf
1 lime, peeled if not organic

Cut produce to fit your juicer's feed tube. Juice all ingredients and stir. Pour into a glass and drink as soon as possible. Serves 1.

Veggie Tonic

1 handful of spinach
1 dark green lettuce leaf
3 ribs of celery with leaves
2 asparagus stems
1 large tomato
1 lemon, peeled if not organic

Cut produce to fit your juicer's feed tube. Wrap spinach in lettuce leaf and push through juicer slowly. Juice remaining ingredients and stir. Pour into a glass and drink as soon as possible. Serves 1.

Very Veggie Rejuvenator

½ tomato
1 cucumber, peeled if not organic
2 carrots, scrubbed well, tops removed, ends trimmed
2 ribs of celery with leaves
1 kale leaf
½ cup green cabbage
1 green onion

Cut produce to fit your juicer's feed tube. Juice all ingredients and stir. Pour into a glass and drink as soon as possible. Serves 2.

Wheatgrass Refresher

1 green apple, washed
1 handful of wheatgrass, rinsed
2–3 sprigs of mint, rinsed (optional)
½ lemon, washed, or peeled if not organic

Cut produce to fit your juicer's feed tube. Start with apple and juice all ingredients and stir. Pour into a glass and drink as soon as possible. Serves 1.

Wheatgrass With Coconut Water

1–2 ounces wheatgrass juice
8 ounces coconut water

Pour wheatgrass juice into a glass. Add coconut water and stir. Serves 1.

Wild Green Energy

1 cucumber, peeled if not organic
1 rib of celery with leaves
1 handful of wild greens such as dandelion,
    nettles, plantain, lamb's quarters, or
    sorrel
1 apple (green is lower in sugar)
1 lemon, peeled if not organic

Cut produce to fit your juicer's feed tube, and push through juicer. Stir and drink as soon as possible. Serves 1.

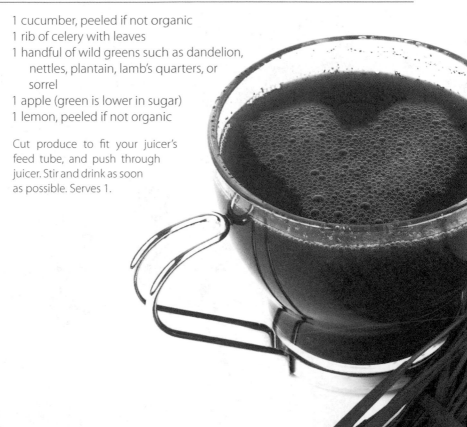

BITTER GREENS

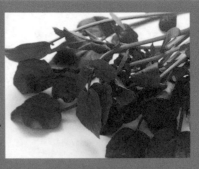

It is believed that bitter greens support the heart, small intestines, and liver, and help reduce fever. As one of the four tastes (alongside sweet, salty, and sour), bitter is now gaining culinary respect. Bitter greens should be one of our choices for juicing as well as cooking. Wild greens reduce the desire for starchy foods, making them an excellent aid in weight loss. The following primer on bitter greens should help you with choosing flavors that combine well with other vegetables and fruit.[2]

- Arugula—the leaves are green or red and oak-shaped; taste is nutty, peppery, and sharp.

- Beet greens—leaves have purple-red veins and bright green flesh; very tangy taste with a hint of mustard and beet flavor.

- Watercress—has small, white-green flowers and is widely available; the taste is hot and sharp.

- Endive—has long, narrow leaves that are white at the base and yellow-green at the tips; the taste is quite bitter.

- Frisee—leaves are short and stiff with curly edges; may be green or blanched with white stems and yellow-green tips; has a mild, slightly bitter flavor.

- Kale—leaves are large, deep green, and curled at the edges; flavor is similar to broccoli, but it has a peppery, bitter finish.

- Mustards—leaves are red or green; taste is sharp and pungent, with a hint of mustard and horseradish.

- Nasturtium—leaves are round and disk-shaped with bright yellow-red-orange flowers; taste is hot and peppery, and it has a hint of horseradish flavor.

- Sorrel—leaves are long and oval-shaped; taste is tart and tangy with a citrus overtone; sorrel was once thought to be poisonous due to its taste.

- Swiss chard—has a broad, fan-shaped green leaf with wide white stems and veins (some have red veins); the taste is mildly bitter.

- Tatsoi—has waxy, round, deep-green leaves; the taste is slightly bitter.

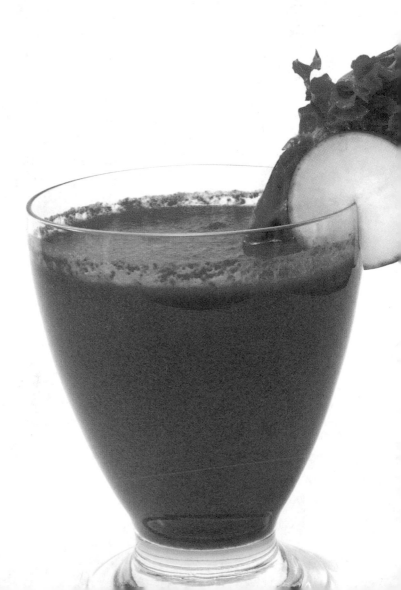

Chapter 5

YUMMY FRUIT JUICE BLENDS

THIS CHAPTER IS filled with delicious fruit juice recipes. This is not what I recommend most people drink every day because these juices contain too much fruit sugar. However, if you are just getting started with juicing, have picky eaters in your family, or children who won't eat or drink their vegetables, this chapter may be a good place to start. These recipes may also be good ones to use when introducing friends to the benefits of juicing. And for babies six months through toddler years, this may be the best place for you to start introducing fresh juices. But keep in mind that you can add one or two green leaves such as kale, chard, collards, or dark green lettuce, and no one will even know it's there. Or you can add some spinach or parsley, and it won't affect the taste. Even for special juice treats, you can add some greens, celery, or a little cucumber, and no one will even suspect that veggies are present. So have fun with this chapter. The juices are yummy!

Apples and Spice

2 apples
1 peach, seeded
¼ tsp. cinnamon or apple-pie spice

Cut produce to fit your juicer's feed tube. Juice all ingredients and stir in spice. Pour into a glass and serve chilled. Serves 1.

Berry Red Refresher

2 slices of watermelon, rind removed if not organic
2 cups of strawberries with caps

Cut produce to fit your juicer's feed tube. Juice all ingredients and stir. Pour into glasses and serve chilled. Serves 2.

Black Currants With Lemons and Apple

2 green apples
½ lemon, peeled if not organic
1 cup fresh black currants

Cut produce to fit your juicer's feed tube. Juice one apple and the lemon. Turn off machine and add currants then the plunger. Turn machine back on and push the currants through. Follow with the second apple and stir the juice. Pour into a glass and serve chilled. Serves 1.

Blackberry Lemonade

2 apples
1 lemon, peeled if not organic
1 cup blackberries, fresh or thawed if frozen

Cut produce to fit your juicer's feed tube. Juice one apple and lemon. Turn off the machine and add the blackberries, then top with the plunger. Turn the machine back on and push berries through; add the remaining apple. Stir the juice and pour into a glass; serve chilled. Serves 1.

Blueberry-Plum-Nectarine-Lemon Cooler

1 plum, pit removed
1 nectarine, peeled, pit removed
1 cup blueberries, fresh or thawed if frozen
1 lemon, peeled if not organic

Cut produce to fit your juicer's feed tube. Juice the plum and nectarine. Turn off the machine and add the blueberries. Top with the plunger. Turn the machine back on and push berries through; then add the lemon. Stir the juice and pour into a glass; serve chilled. Serves 1.

Cantaloupe-Mint Cooler

½ cantaloupe, with seeds and rind if organic
6 sprigs of fresh mint

Cut produce to fit your juicer's feed tube. Juice all ingredients and stir. Pour into a glass and serve immediately. Serves 1.

Cranberry-Pear-Apple Cocktail

1 red delicious or other sweet apple
¼ cup cranberries, fresh or thawed if frozen
1 pear (Asian or Bartlett)
1 small piece fresh beet for color (optional)

Cut produce to fit your juicer's feed tube. Juice the apple. Turn off the machine and add the cranberries. Top with the plunger. Turn the machine back on and push berries through; then add the pear and beet (if using). Stir the juice and pour into a glass; serve chilled. Serves 1.

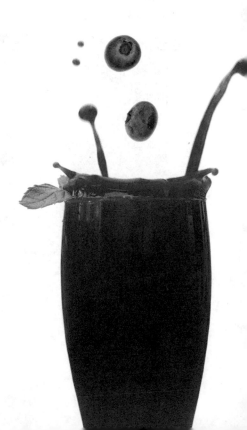

Elderberry-Strawberry-Apple Cocktail

1 apple
1 cup elderberries
1 cup strawberries with caps

Cut produce to fit your juicer's feed tube. Juice the apple. Turn off the machine and add the elderberries. Top with the plunger. Turn the machine back on and push berries through; then add the strawberries. Stir the juice and pour into a glass; serve chilled. Serves 1.

Fruit Punch

2 apples
¼ honeydew melon with rind if organic
1 cup red grapes
½ lemon, peeled if not organic
1-inch-chunk ginger root

Cut produce to fit your juicer's feed tube. Juice all ingredients and stir. Pour into a glass and drink as soon as possible. Serves 2.

Grapefruit-Strawberry Sparkler

1 grapefruit, peeled
1 lime, peeled if not organic
10 strawberries with caps
1 cup chilled sparkling water

Cut produce to fit your juicer's feed tube. Juice all ingredients and stir in sparkling water. Pour into a glass and served chilled. Serves 2.

Hawaiian Breeze

1 orange, peeled
¼ fresh pineapple, peeled if not organic
½ cup coconut water

Cut produce to fit your juicer's feed tube. Juice all ingredients and stir in the coconut water. Pour into a glass and serve chilled. Serves 1.

Honeydew Limeade

½ honeydew melon, with seeds and rind removed if not organic
1 lime, peeled if not organic
½ apple

Cut produce to fit your juicer's feed tube. Juice all ingredients and stir. Pour into a glass and serve chilled. Serves 1–2.

Island Punch

1 orange, peeled
¼ pineapple, peeled if not organic
1 lime, peeled if not organic
Dash of freshly grated nutmeg to taste

Cut produce to fit your juicer's feed tube. Juice all ingredients, then stir in nutmeg. Pour into a glass and serve chilled. Serves 1–2.

Key Lime Cooler

2 apples
1 lime, peeled if not organic

Cut produce to fit your juicer's feed tube. Juice all ingredients and stir. Pour into a glass over ice and serve. Serves 1.

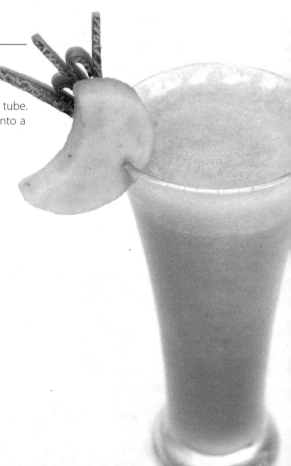

Kumquat-Grape-Kiwi-Orange Cocktail

6 kumquats, with peel
3 kiwifruit, with peel
1 orange, peeled
1 lemon, peeled if not organic
1 small bunch of black grapes (you can include small stems)

Cut produce to fit your juicer's feed tube. Juice all ingredients and stir. Pour into a glass and serve chilled. Serves 1–2.

Lemon-Lime Slushy

Juice of two limes, peeled if not organic
Juice of one lemon, peeled if not organic
4–6 drops stevia
1½ cups sparkling water
Ice

Mix the juice with the stevia and sparkling water. Pour into two tall glasses over ice and drink as soon as possible. Serves 2.

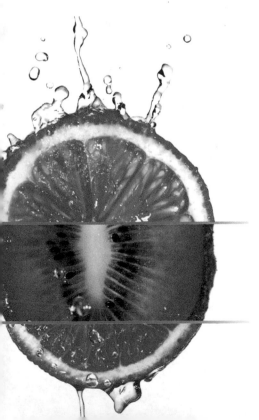

Lemon-Lime-Blueberry Refresher

1 cucumber, peeled if not organic
1 apple
1 cup blueberries, fresh or thawed if frozen
½ lemon, peeled if not organic
½ lime, peeled if not organic

Cut produce to fit your juicer's feed tube. Juice the cucumber and apple. Turn off the machine and add the blueberries. Top with the plunger. Turn the machine back on and push berries through; then juice the lemon and lime. Stir the juice and pour into a glass; serve chilled. Serves 1.

Lime-Apple-Mint Cocktail

2 apples
1 lime, peeled if not organic
1 small handful of mint

Cut produce to fit your juicer's feed tube. Juice all ingredients and stir. Pour into a glass and serve chilled. Serves 1.

Mango Limeade

2 apples
1 lime, peeled if not organic
1 mango, peeled and seeded

Cut produce to fit your juicer's feed tube. Juice all ingredients and stir. Pour into a glass and serve chilled. Serves 1.

Mango-Watercress Refresher

1 mango, peeled and seeded
½ cucumber, peeled if not organic
1 handful of watercress

Cut produce to fit your juicer's feed tube. Juice all ingredients and stir. Pour into a glass and serve chilled. Serves 1.

Melon-Pineapple-Lemon-Mint Cocktail

½ cantaloupe with seeds, peeled if not organic
¼ pineapple, peeled if not organic
1 handful of fresh mint
1 dark green lettuce leaf
1 lemon, peeled if not organic

Cut produce to fit your juicer's feed tube. Juice all ingredients and stir. Pour into a glass and serve chilled. Serves 1.

Mint Lemonade

2 apples
1 lemon, peeled if not organic
1 small handful of mint

Cut produce to fit your juicer's feed tube. Juice all ingredients and stir. Pour into a glass and serve chilled. Serves 1.

Mixed Berry Delight

2 green apples
1 lemon, peeled if not organic
2 cups mixed berries such as blackberries, raspberries, and blueberries

Cut produce to fit your juicer's feed tube. Juice one apple and lemon. Turn off the machine and add the berries. Top with the plunger. Turn the machine back on and push berries through; then juice the remaining apple. Stir the juice and pour into a glass; serve chilled. Serves 1.

Orange-Apple Fizz

1 cup fresh apple juice (about 2 apples)
1 cup fresh orange juice (about 2 oranges)
1 cup sparkling water

Juice the apples and oranges to make 1 cup of juice for each. Stir in the sparkling water. Pour into glasses over ice and serve chilled. Serves 2.

Orange-Apricot Delight

2 oranges, peeled
1 apricot, pit removed
1 lime, peeled if not organic

Cut produce to fit your juicer's feed tube. Juice all ingredients and stir. Pour into a glass and serve chilled. Serves 1.

Orange-Berry Blaster

2 oranges, peeled
1 cup berries, such as raspberries, blackberries, or blueberries
1 kiwifruit

Cut produce to fit your juicer's feed tube. Juice one orange. Turn off machine, add berries, and put the plunger in place. Turn the machine back on and push the berries through. Follow with the other orange and kiwifruit. Stir the juice. Pour into a glass and serve chilled. Serves 1–2.

Orange-Lemon-Ginger Cooler

2 oranges, peeled
1 lemon, peeled if not organic
1-inch-chunk ginger root

Cut produce to fit your juicer's feed tube. Juice all ingredients and stir. Pour into a glass over ice and serve. Serves 1–2.

Orange-Spinach Refresher

2 oranges, peeled
1 handful of spinach
1 rib of celery with leaves

Cut produce to fit your juicer's feed tube. Juice all ingredients and stir. Pour into a glass and serve chilled. Serves 1.

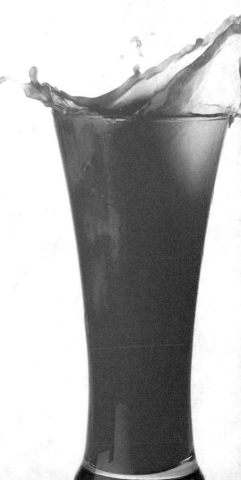

Peach-Blackberry-Apple Cocktail

1 peach, pit removed
1 cup blackberries, fresh or thawed if frozen
1 apple

Cut produce to fit your juicer's feed tube. Juice peach. Turn off machine, add blackberries, then put the plunger in place. Turn the machine back on and push the berries through. Follow with the apple and stir the juice. Pour into a glass and serve chilled. Serves 1.

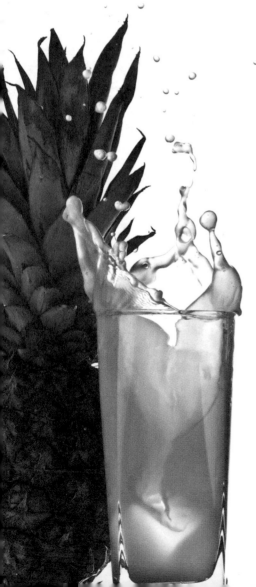

Pear-Ginger-Currant Cocktail

1 apple
1 pear
1 cup fresh currants
1-inch-chunk fresh ginger root
½ lemon, peeled if not organic

Cut produce to fit your juicer's feed tube. Juice apple and pear. Turn off machine, add currants, then put the plunger in place. Turn machine back on and push the currants through. Follow with the ginger root and lemon; stir the juice. Pour into a glass and serve chilled. Serves 1.

Pear-Kiwi-Mint Delight

1 pear
1 kiwifruit with skin
1 small handful of mint

Cut produce to fit your juicer's feed tube. Juice all ingredients and stir. Pour into a glass and serve chilled. Serves 1.

Perky Pear-Apple Cocktail

1 pear
1 apple
1-inch-chunk ginger root

Cut produce to fit your juicer's feed tube. Juice all ingredients and stir. Pour into a glass and serve chilled. Serves 1.

Pineapple Lemonade

2 apples
1 lemon, peeled if not organic
¼ pineapple, peeled if not organic

Cut produce to fit your juicer's feed tube. Juice all ingredients and stir. Pour into a glass and serve chilled. Serves 1.

Pineapple Mint Cooler

1 apple
¼ pineapple, peeled if not organic
1 small handful of mint
1 cup chilled sparkling water

Cut produce to fit your juicer's feed tube. Juice all ingredients and stir in sparkling water. Pour into glasses and serve chilled. Serves 2.

Pineapple Mint Delight

¼ pineapple, peeled if not organic
1 handful of fresh mint

Cut produce to fit your juicer's feed tube. Juice all ingredients and stir. Pour into a glass and serve chilled. Serves 1.

Pineapple-Carrot Nectar

¼ fresh pineapple, peeled if not organic
3 carrots, scrubbed well, tops removed, ends trimmed
1 green apple

Cut produce to fit your juicer's feed tube. Juice all ingredients and stir. Pour into a glass and serve chilled. Serves 1.

Pineapple-Ginger Sparkler

¼ pineapple, peeled if not organic
1-inch-chunk ginger root
½ cup sparkling water, chilled

Cut produce to fit your juicer's feed tube. Juice all ingredients and stir in sparkling water. Pour into a glass and serve chilled. Serves 1.

Pineapple-Orange Refresher

2 oranges, peeled
¼ pineapple, peeled if not organic
½ lemon, peeled if not organic

Cut produce to fit your juicer's feed tube. Juice all ingredients and stir. Pour into a glass and serve chilled. Serves 1–2.

Pink Lemonade Sparkler

2 apples
1 lemon, peeled if not organic
¼ beet with leaves
1 cup chilled sparkling water

Cut produce to fit your juicer's feed tube. Juice all ingredients and stir in sparkling water. Pour into a glass and serve chilled. Serves 1–2.

Plain Janie

1 apple
1 cup strawberries with caps

Cut produce to fit your juicer's feed tube. Juice all ingredients and stir. Pour into a glass and serve chilled. Serves 1.

Plum Lemonade

2 apples
2 ripe red or black plums, pits removed
1 lemon, peeled if not organic

Cut produce to fit your juicer's feed tube. Juice all ingredients and stir. Pour into a glass and serve chilled. Serves 1–2.

Plum-Honeydew-Tarragon

½ honeydew melon with seeds, rind removed if not organic
1 plum, seed removed
3 sprigs of fresh tarragon

Cut produce to fit your juicer's feed tube. Juice all ingredients and stir. Pour into a glass and serve chilled. Serves 1–2.

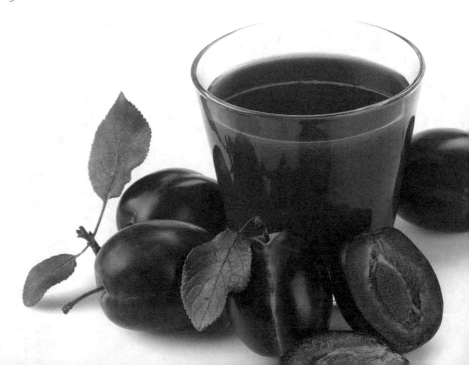

Plum-Orange-Mint Cooler

2 oranges, peeled
1 plum, seeded
1 small handful of mint

Cut produce to fit your juicer's feed tube. Juice all ingredients and stir. Pour into a glass and serve chilled. Serves 1.

Pom Pom

2 pomegranates
2 apples
½ lemon, peeled if not organic
1-inch-chunk ginger root

Cut the pomegranates in half. Pull the skin away and remove the seeds. Place the clusters of seeds in a bowl. Cut the apples to fit your juicer's feed tube. Pour about one-third of the pomegranate seeds in the juicer with the machine turned off, then put the plunger in place. Turn the machine on and push the pomegranate seeds through. Follow with apple chunks and keep alternating the apple and 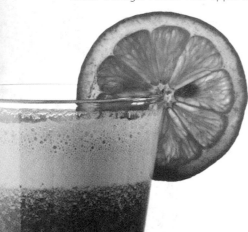 pomegranate seeds until all the seeds have been juiced. Always turn machine off when juicing seeds, or they will fly out. Follow with the lemon, ginger, and any remaining apple. Stir and drink as soon as possible. Serves 1.

Raspberry Limeade

2 apples
1 lime, peeled if not organic
1 cup raspberries

Cut produce to fit your juicer's feed tube. Juice one apple and lime. Turn off the machine and add the raspberries. Top with the plunger. Turn the machine back on and push berries through; add the remaining apple. Stir the juice and pour into a glass; serve chilled. Serves 1.

Raspberry-Orange Lemonade

1 orange, peeled
1 cup raspberries
2 apples
1 lemon, peeled if not organic

Cut produce to fit your juicer's feed tube. Juice orange. Turn off the machine and add the raspberries. Top with the plunger. Turn the machine back on and push berries through; then juice the remaining ingredients. Stir the juice and pour into a glass; serve chilled. Serves 2.

Razz and Spazz

1 apple
1 cup raspberries, fresh or thawed if frozen
½ cucumber, peeled if not organic
¼ cup fresh mint leaves

Cut produce to fit your juicer's feed tube. Juice one apple. Turn off the machine and add the raspberries. Top with the plunger. Turn the machine back on and push berries through; then add the remaining apple, cucumber, and mint. Stir the juice and pour into a glass; serve chilled. Serves 1.

Red, White, and Blue

1 cup cranberries or raspberries, fresh or thawed if frozen
1 cup blueberries, fresh or thawed if frozen
1 small bunch of white grapes (you can juice small stems)

Pour berries into the juicer while it is off and top with the plunger, or the berries will fly out. Push berries through then add the grapes. Stir the juice and pour into a glass; serve chilled. Serves 1.

Romaine-Orange-Apple Refresher

1 orange, peeled
1 green apple
3–4 romaine lettuce leaves

Cut produce to fit your juicer's feed tube. Juice all ingredients and stir. Pour into a glass and serve chilled. Serves 1.

Rosy Girl

½ pineapple with core, peeled if not organic
1 cup strawberries, fresh with caps or thawed if frozen
¼ small beet with leaves

Cut produce to fit your juicer's feed tube. Juice all ingredients and stir. Pour into a glass and serve chilled. Serves 1.

Spicy Cantaloupe Refresher

½ ripe cantaloupe with seeds, peel removed
½ cucumber, peeled if not organic
1 kale leaf
1 lime, peeled if not organic
1- to 2-inch-chunk ginger root, peeled

Cut produce to fit your juicer's feed tube. Juice all ingredients and stir. Pour into a glass and serve chilled. Serves 1.

Strawberry Bliss

2 peaches, seeded
2 cups strawberries, fresh with caps or thawed if frozen
1-inch-chunk ginger root

Cut produce to fit your juicer's feed tube. Juice all ingredients and stir. Pour into a glass and serve chilled. Serves 1.

Strawberry-Mint Cordial

1 pint fresh strawberries with caps
1 handful of mint
1–2 drops stevia
1 cup sparkling water

Juice the strawberries and mint. Pour in a glass and add the stevia and sparkling water. Stir and serve over ice. Serves 1.

Strawberry-Rhubarb Lemonade

10–12 fresh strawberries with caps
2–3 stalks rhubarb, without leaves (the leaves are toxic)
2 apples
1 lemon, peeled if not organic
1–2 drops stevia (optional)

Cut produce to fit your juicer's feed tube. Juice all ingredients and stir in stevia as desired. Pour into a glass and serve chilled. Serves 1.

Summer Cooler

2 slices watermelon, about 2–3 inches wide by 5 inches long, rind removed
    if not organic
1 lime, peeled if not organic

Cut produce to fit your juicer's feed tube. Juice all ingredients. Pour into ice-filled glasses and serve chilled. Serves 2.

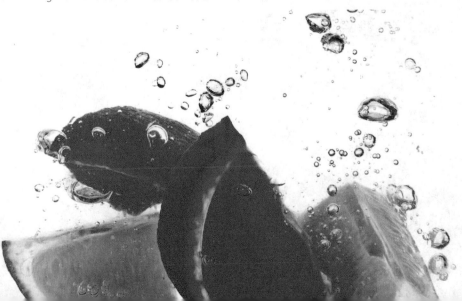

Sweet Apricot-Apple-Mint Cocktail

2 green apples
2 apricots, pits removed
1 small handful of mint

Cut produce to fit your juicer's feed tube. Juice all ingredients and stir. Pour into a glass and served chilled. Serves 1.

Sweet Basil Lemonade

2 apples
1 lemon, peeled if not organic
1 small handful of fresh basil

Cut produce to fit your juicer's feed tube. Juice all ingredients and stir. Pour into a glass and serve chilled. Serves 1.

Tangerine Sparkler

4 tangerines, peeled
1 cup chilled sparkling water

Juice tangerines and stir in sparkling water. Serve chilled. Serves 1.

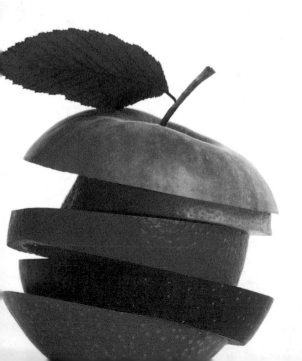

Watermelon-Cranberry Cooler

1 cup cranberries, fresh or thawed if frozen
⅛ small watermelon, with rind if organic, cut in strips to fit your juicer
½ lime, peeled if not organic

Pour cranberries in juicer with machine turned off. Top with plunger. Turn on machine and push berries through, followed by watermelon and lime. Sir and pour into glasses. Serve chilled. Serves 2.

White Grape-Tangerine Cocktail

4 tangerines, peeled
1 small bunch of white grapes (you can juice small stems)
½ green apple

Cut produce to fit your juicer's feed tube. Juice all ingredients and stir. Pour into a glass and serve chilled. Serves 1.

Zesty Morning

1 pink grapefruit, peeled
2 oranges, peeled
1 lime, peeled if not organic
1-inch-chunk ginger root

Cut produce to fit your juicer's feed tube. Juice all ingredients and stir. Pour into a glass and serve chilled. Serves 2.

Chapter 6

OLD FAVORITES

THIS CHAPTER OFFERS many of my favorite juice recipes that have become very popular over the years. These recipes appeared in my books *The Juice Lady's Turbo Diet* and *The Juice Lady's Living Foods Revolution*. If you're looking for meal plans for weight loss and lots of tips for losing weight, get *The Juice Lady's Turbo Diet*. If you're looking for a very informative basic book to give you general meal plans and lots of raw food recipes, get *The Juice Lady's Living Foods Revolution*. These books are great companions to *The Juice Lady's Big Book of Juices and Green Smoothies*.

Whether you try the "old favorite" juice recipes in this chapter or any of the hundreds of new recipes in this book, I think you'll be amazed at what a juicing program can do for your health. Here's what it has done for Joann:

> I just got your book *The Juice Lady's Living Foods Revolution* after talking with my friend, who told me how she is continuously feeling better and better and how good her skin looks after eating and drinking according to your book. Before getting your book, I watched the documentary *Forks Over Knives*, which is about animal fats (meats and dairy) that have a direct impact on the prevalence of cancer and other diseases. It turned me off to bad foods. I decided to stop eating most meats and cut out as much dairy as possible. I started eating more vegan and including more raw foods.
>
> It was hard for me to change eating habits initially and to find recipes. Then I remembered *The Juice Lady's*

Living Foods Revolution that my friend spoke about. It took a while for my husband to order your book and the juicer, so in the meantime I used my blender to make green smoothies. I had one for breakfast and took two to work every day. For regular meals I ate somewhat normally but cut out meat. I still eat fish and a little chicken and dairy occasionally, with plenty of vegetables, fruits, whole-grain pasta (if I eat pasta, which is not very often), and brown rice instead of white rice. Now that I have the juicer, I have a vegetable juice first thing in the morning, and I take two green smoothies to work.

After about a month I've lost eight pounds! This was an unexpected benefit. Weight loss was not my primary goal, but it's a very welcome one. And I lost this weight without working out because I haven't had time lately. I assume that when I get back in the swing of working out regularly, I will lose weight even faster.

Beet, Carrot, Coconut Blast

4–5 carrots, scrubbed well, tops removed, ends trimmed
1 small beet with leaves
½–1 cup coconut milk
Dash cayenne pepper

Juice the carrots and beet. Pour into a glass and add the coconut milk and cayenne pepper. Stir and drink as soon as possible. Serves 2.

Carrot and Spice

2–3 carrots, scrubbed well, tops
    removed, ends trimmed
1 handful of spinach
1 cucumber, peeled if not organic
½ lemon, peeled if not organic
½ apple (green has less sugar)
1-inch-chunk ginger root
¼ tsp. cinnamon
⅛ tsp. cayenne pepper

Cut produce to fit your juicer's feed tube. Juice all ingredients. Add spices and stir. Pour the juice into two glasses, and drink as soon as possible. Serves 2.

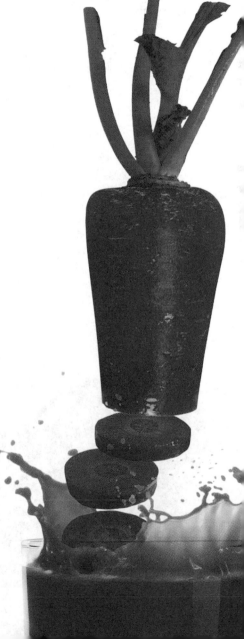

Cranberry-Pear Fat Buster

Studies show that cranberries boost metabolism and their acids help dissolve fat. They also act as a diuretic, which helps you get rid of stored up water. The credit goes to their soluble fiber, which is not lost entirely with juicing.

2 pears, Bartlett or Asian
½ cucumber, peeled if not organic
¼ lemon, peeled if not organic
2 tablespoons cranberries, fresh or thawed if frozen
½- to 1-inch-chunk ginger root

Cut produce to fit your juicer's feed tube. With the juicer turned off, add the cranberries and top with the plunger. Then turn on your machine and juice. Juice all remaining ingredients and stir. Pour into a glass and drink as soon as possible. Serves 1.

Energize-Your-Day Cocktail

1 apple (green is lower in sugar)
2 dark green leaves (chard, collard, or kale)
1 rib of celery with leaves
1 lemon, peeled if not organic
½ cucumber, peeled if not organic
½- to 1-inch-chunk fresh ginger root, peeled

Cut the apple into sections that fit your juicer's feed tube. Roll the green leaves and push through the feed tube with the apple, celery, lemon, cucumber, and ginger. Stir the juice and pour into a glass. Drink as soon as possible. Serves 1.

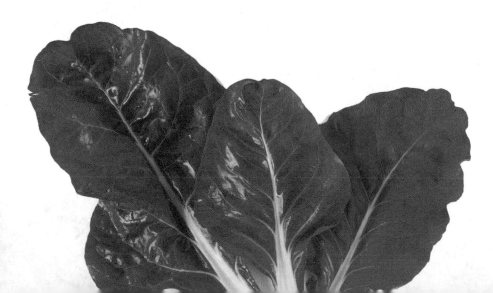

Green Berry Blast

1 cucumber, peeled if not organic
4 dark green leaves such as collard, chard, or kale
1 cup blueberries, fresh or thawed if frozen
1 apple (green is lower in sugar)
½ lemon, peeled if not organic

Cut produce to fit your juicer's feed tube. Juice half of the cucumber. Roll the green leaves and push through the juicer with the other half of the cucumber. Turn off the machine and pour in the berries, then place the plunger on top. Turn the machine on and push the berries through. Add the apple and lemon, and juice. Stir the juice and drink as soon as possible. Serves 2.

Green Lemonade

2 apples (green is lower in sugar)
½ lemon, peeled if not organic
1 handful of your favorite greens

Cut product to fit your juicer's feed tube. Juice all ingredients and stir. Pour into a glass and drink as soon as possible. Serves 1.

Happy-Mood Morning

Fennel juice has been used as a traditional tonic to help the body release endorphins, the "feel-good" peptides, from the brain into the bloodstream. Endorphins help to diminish anxiety and fear, and they generate a mood of euphoria.

½ apple (green is lower in sugar)
4–5 carrots, well scrubbed, tops removed, ends trimmed
3 fennel stalks with leaves and flowers
½ cucumber, peeled if not organic
1 handful of spinach
1-inch-chunk ginger root

Cut produce to fit your juicer's feed tube. Juice apple first and follow with other ingredients. Stir and pour into a glass; drink as soon as possible. Serves 1–2.

Jicama Surprise

2-inch by 4- or 5-inch chunk of jicama, scrubbed well or peeled if not
    organic
2–3 carrots, scrubbed well, tops removed, ends trimmed
½ cucumber, peeled if not organic
¼ daikon radish, trimmed and scrubbed
1-inch-chunk ginger root, scrubbed (peel if old)
½ lemon or lime, peeled if not organic

Cut produce to fit your juicer's feed tube. Juice ingredients and stir. Pour into a
glass and drink as soon as possible. Serves 1.

Peppy Parsley

1 cucumber, peeled if not organic
1 carrot, scrubbed well, tops removed, ends trimmed
1 rib of celery with leaves
1 handful of parsley
1 kale leaf
1 lemon, peeled if not organic

Cut produce to fit your juicer's feed tube. Juice cucumber, carrot, and celery.
Bunch up the parsley and roll in the kale leaf; add to juicer and push through.
Then add lemon and juice. Stir and pour into a glass. Drink as soon as possible.
Serves 1.

Raging Beet-Jalapeño

1 beet with tops
2 collard or Swiss chard leaves
1 cucumber, peeled if not organic
1 lemon, peeled if not organic
1-inch-chunk ginger root
⅛–¼ small jalapeño pepper, seeds removed

Cut produce to fit your juicer's feed tube. Juice the beet with tops. Roll collard
or chard leaves and follow with ½ cucumber. Add other ingredients and follow
with the remaining cucumber. Pour juice into a glass, stir, and drink as soon as
possible. Serves 1.

Spicy Pink Morning

1 large pink grapefruit, peeled
1-inch-chunk fresh ginger root

Cut produce to fit your juicer's feed tube. Juice ingredients and stir. Pour into a glass and drink as soon as possible. Serves 1.

Spring Veggie Tonic

Asparagus is a natural diuretic that helps flush toxins from the body and promotes kidney cleansing. This juice is a great tonic for the kidneys, and it is a great way to use up asparagus stems.

1 tomato
1 cucumber, peeled if not organic
8 asparagus stems
1 lemon, peeled if not organic

Cut produce to fit your juicer's feed tube. Juice all ingredients and stir. Pour into a glass and drink as soon as possible. Serves 1–2.

The Ginger Hopper With a Twist

5 medium carrots, scrubbed well, tops removed, ends trimmed
1 green apple
1-inch-chunk fresh ginger root, peeled
½ lemon, peeled if not organic

Cut produce to fit your juicer's feed tube. Juice ingredients and stir. Pour into a glass and drink as soon as possible. Serves 1.

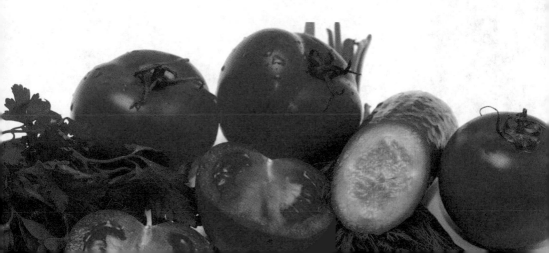

The Morning Energizer

4 carrots, scrubbed well, tops removed, ends trimmed
1 handful of parsley
1 lemon, peeled if not organic
1 apple (green has less sugar)
2-inch-chunk fresh ginger root, peeled

Cut produce to fit your juicer's feed tube. Juice ingredients and stir. Pour into a glass and drink as soon as possible. Serves 1.

The Waldorf

1 green apple
3 ribs of celery with leaves
1 lemon, peeled if not organic

Cut produce to fit your juicer's feed tube. Juice ingredients and stir. Pour into a glass and drink as soon as possible. Serves 1.

Tomato and Spice

2 medium tomatoes
2 dark green leaves
2 radishes
Small handful of parsley
1 lime or lemon, peeled if not organic
Dash of hot sauce

Cut produce to fit your juicer's feed tube. Juice ingredients, add hot sauce, and stir. Pour into a glass and drink as soon as possible. Serves 1.

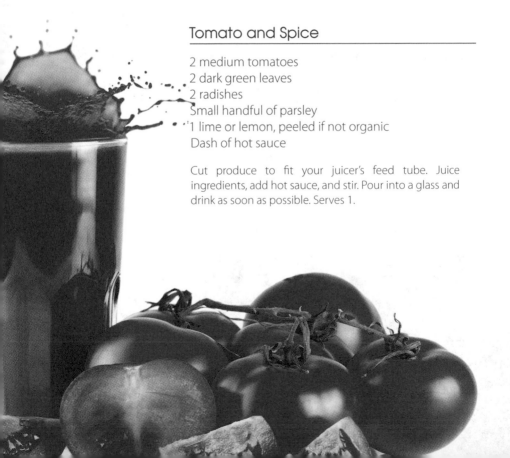

Tomato Florentine

2 tomatoes
4–5 sprigs of basil
1 large handful of spinach
1 lemon, peeled if not organic

Juice one tomato. Wrap the basil in several spinach leaves. Turn off the machine and add the spinach and basil. Turn the machine back on and gently tap to juice them. Juice the remaining tomato and lemon. Stir juice, pour in a glass, and drink as soon as possible. Serves 1.

Veggie Time

4 carrots, scrubbed well, tops removed, ends trimmed
1 turnip, scrubbed well
1 lemon, peeled if not organic
2-inch-chunk jicama, scrubbed or peeled if not organic
1 handful of watercress
1 garlic clove

Cut produce to fit your juicer's feed tube. Juice all ingredients and stir. Pour into a glass and drink as soon as possible. Serves 1–2.

Weight-Loss Buddy

Jerusalem artichoke juice combined with carrot and beet is a traditional remedy for satisfying cravings for sweets and junk food. The key is to sip this juice slowly when you get a craving for high-fat or high-carb foods.

3–4 carrots, scrubbed well, tops removed, ends trimmed
1 Jerusalem artichoke, scrubbed well
1 cucumber, peeled if not organic
1 lemon, peeled if not organic
½ small beet, with stems and leaves, scrubbed well

Cut produce to fit your juicer's feed tube. Juice ingredients and stir. Pour into a glass and drink as soon as possible. Serves 1.

You Are Loved Cocktail

3 carrots, scrubbed well, tops removed, ends trimmed
2 ribs of celery with leaves
1 cucumber, peeled if not organic
1 handful of spinach
1 lemon, peeled if not organic
½ beet, scrubbed well, with stems and leaves

Cut produce to fit your juicer's feed tube. Juice all ingredients and stir. Pour into a glass and drink as soon as possible. Serves 1–2.

WANT TO LOSE WEIGHT? ALKALIZE YOUR BODY

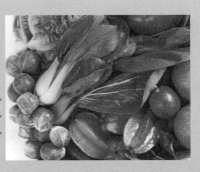

Many people eat a high-sugar breakfast consisting of foods such as orange juice, toast, jam, honey, sweetened cereal, sweet rolls, doughnuts, muffins, waffles, or pancakes. All this sugar promotes acidity and causes yeast and fungus to grow, which produces acid. An overly acidic condition can cause you to gain weight and not be able to lose it. But avoiding sugar and simple carbohydrates alone isn't the answer. Traditional high-protein breakfast foods such as omelets, cheese, bacon, sausage, and meat promote elevated acid levels in the body as well. Add to that highly acidic drinks such as coffee, black tea, soda pop, alcohol, and sports drinks, and you can see how much acid-forming food people consume throughout the day.

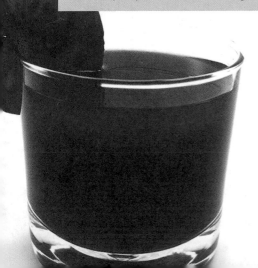

Keep in mind that when I call something acid-forming, I am not necessarily referring to the state it is in when you eat or drink it. I am referring to the fact that after these kinds of foods are metabolized, they leave an ash residue. As a result of eating acid-forming foods, coupled with not eating enough greens and other living foods, many people suffer from a condition known as mild acidosis, which is an out-of-balance pH that leans toward acidity. This means the body is continually fighting to maintain pH balance.

One of the symptoms of acidosis is weight gain and an inability to lose the weight. (This often exacerbates another symptom of acidosis—joint and muscle pain.) The reason is that the body tends to store acid in fat cells and hang on to those cells to protect its delicate tissues and organs. It will even make more fat cells in which to store acid if they're needed. To turn this scenario around, it's important to alkalize your body. Eating greens is one of the best ways to do that, and juicing gives you an easy way to consume a lot more greens than you could chew in a day.

To give your body a great start in rebalancing your pH, make sure 60 percent to 80 percent of your diet is made up of alkalizing foods such as green vegetables, raw juices, grasses such as wheatgrass, fresh fruit and vegetables, raw seeds and nuts, and sprouts. Greatly limit or avoid your consumption of acid-forming foods such as meat, dairy products, chocolate, sweets, bread and all other yeast products, alcohol, carbonated drinks, sports drinks, coffee, and black tea.

When pH balance is achieved, the body should automatically drop to its ideal, healthy weight unless you have other health challenges. (But those should heal too over time.) As the acidic environment is neutralized with mineral-rich alkaline foods, there will be no need for your body to create new fat cells to store acid. And since the remaining fat is no longer needed to store acid wastes, it simply melts away.

Eating alkalizing foods is also a great way to restore your health. Many diseases such as cancer thrive in an acidic state. Take away the acid, and they don't do as well. An alkaline diet also boosts your energy level, improves skin, reduces allergies, sustains the immune system, and enhances mental clarity.

Chapter 7

JUICE REMEDIES AND REJUVENATORS

O VER AND OVER in my practice as a nutritionist I've witnessed the healing power of fresh juice. Since I wrote my first juice book, *Juicing for Life*, in 1991, I've sold more than three million books on juicing. Currently my most popular book on juice remedies, *The Juice Lady's Guide to Juicing for Health*, covers more than fifty different ailments and the juice therapies that, along with diet, supplements, and lifestyle changes, may help heal those conditions.

This chapter covering juice remedies and rejuvenators will help get you started on the road to healing and rejuvenation. If you want to do more to heal your body, get my companion guide *The Juice Lady's Guide to Juicing for Health*, which gives you the complete program of diet, supplements, and lifestyle changes needed for the particular condition you're dealing with. Do juice remedies really help in healing the body? I'd like to share with you Ann's story. She's one of thousands of people who have experienced the healing power of juicing.

About nineteen years ago Ann was diagnosed with lung sarcoidosis, which involves inflammation and is characterized by the formation of tiny lumps of cells (granulomas) in the lungs. She had difficulty breathing, very little energy to accomplish things, and vertigo. She also developed a polyp in her sinuses. She took antibiotics because her doctors thought she had a bacterial infection, but the antibiotics didn't help her. Then one day she sensed God was directing her to eat and drink a "living foods diet" as explained in my books *The Juice Lady's Turbo Diet* and *The Juice Lady's Living Foods Revolution*.

She believed that after making this change in her diet and lifestyle, she would be healed.

With nothing to lose, she embarked on a three-month program of living foods and juices. To her amazement she stopped feeling tired and weak, and her breathing improved. As long as she stuck with the raw foods and vegetable juices, she felt good every day. If she cheated, even a little, she felt sick, like she had a food hangover in the morning. One day a relative persuaded her to have half a glass of wine. She felt really sick the next day and knew she couldn't cheat again. This live-foods program had to be her way of life.

Ann said amazing things are happening in her body. For example, she had a "dent" in her head, with a knot or raised area in the middle. Now the dent is filling in and the knot is shrinking. Recently she put on her "skinny jeans" and realized that her thighs were smaller and the jeans fit very well. But the best part is that her lungs are healing. Though they are not completely healed, they are improving with each day. Can she stick with this diet? I love how she answered: "Nothing tastes as good as great health!" I hope the following recipes will help set you on a path toward great health too.

Adrenal Booster

Hot peppers and parsley are rich in vitamin C; celery is a great source of natural sodium. Both are very beneficial for the adrenal glands.

1 handful of parsley
1 dark green lettuce leaf
4 carrots, scrubbed well, tops removed, ends trimmed
2 tomatoes
2 ribs of celery with leaves
Dash of hot sauce
Dash of Celtic sea salt

Cut produce to fit your juicer's feed tube. Wrap the parsley in the lettuce leaf and push through the juicer slowly. Juice all remaining ingredients, add hot sauce and sea salt, and stir. Pour into a glass and drink as soon as possible. Serves 2.

Allergy Remedy

Parsley is a known "folk remedy" for allergy attacks. This juice recipe once saved my husband after an allergic reaction to walnuts. I never discount folk remedies.

1 large bunch of parsley
¼–½ small or medium lemon, washed or peeled if not organic
2–3 carrots, scrubbed well, tops removed, ends trimmed
2 ribs of celery with leaves
1 cucumber, peeled if not organic

Cut produce to fit your juicer's feed tube. Bunch up parsley and add to the juicer before turning it on. Then add lemon and place the plunger in place. Turn on the machine and juice remaining ingredients. Stir and pour into a glass. Drink as soon as possible. Serves 1.

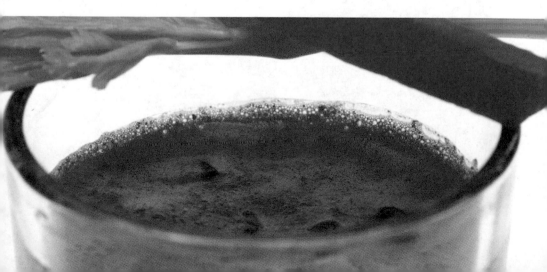

Antiaging Rejuvenator

Cucumber and bell pepper are good sources of the trace mineral silicon, which is recommended to firm up the skin. Silicon has been shown to reduce signs of aging, including improving skin thickness and reducing wrinkles.

1 cucumber, peeled if not organic
1 parsnip
2–3 carrots, scrubbed well, tops removed, ends trimmed
½ lemon, peeled if not organic
¼ green bell pepper with seeds and membrane

Cut produce to fit your juicer's feed tube. Juice ingredients and stir. Pour into a glass and drink as soon as possible. Serves 1–2.

Antianxiety Cocktail

As I stated in chapter 4, magnesium is known as "nature's Valium." If you're prone to anxiety attacks, include plenty of magnesium-rich veggies such as beet leaves, spinach, parsley, dandelion greens, broccoli, cauliflower, carrots, and celery in your juices.

3–4 carrots, scrubbed well, tops removed, ends trimmed
2 ribs of celery with leaves
1 handful of spinach
1 dark green lettuce leaf
1 broccoli stem
1 lemon, peeled if not organic

Cut produce to fit your juicer's feed tube. Juice all ingredients and stir. Pour into a glass and drink as soon as possible. Serves 1.

Arthritis Helper

Ginger has anti-inflammatory properties that can help reduce arthritic joint pain and help combat oxidative damage to joints.

1 handful of flat-leaf parsley
1 dark green lettuce leaf
3–4 carrots, scrubbed well, tops removed, ends trimmed
2 ribs of celery with leaves
2-inch-chunk ginger root
1 lemon, peeled if not organic

Cut produce to fit your juicer's feed tube. Wrap the parsley in the lettuce leaf and push through the juicer slowly. Juice all remaining ingredients and stir. Pour into a glass and drink as soon as possible. Serves 1.

Asthma Helper

Radish is a traditional remedy for asthma.

5 carrots, scrubbed well, tops removed, ends trimmed
5–6 radishes with leaves
1 green apple
½ lemon, peeled if not organic

Cut produce to fit your juicer's feed tube. Juice all ingredients. Stir and pour into a glass. Serve at room temperature or chilled, as desired. Serves 1.

Berry Bright Eyes

Berries are very rich in antioxidants that help fight degenerative eye disorders. They also help improve vision. You can also help prevent eye disorders by avoiding sugar. Eating too much sugar promotes swelling of the lenses and increases the risk of free-radical damage to the eyes.

1 Wild Berry Zinger herbal tea bag
½ cup blackberries, fresh or thawed if frozen
½ cup blueberries, fresh or thawed if frozen
1 handful of spinach
1 dark green lettuce leaf
¼ tsp. pure raspberry extract

Steep one bag of Wild Berry Zinger herbal tea in a cup of hot water for about twenty minutes, or until the tea is strong and flavorful. Set aside to cool. With the juicer off pour in the berries. Turn the machine on and juice the berries. Then wrap spinach in the lettuce leaf and push through the juicer slowly. Juice all remaining ingredients and combine with herbal tea and raspberry extract. Stir and serve as soon as possible. Serves 1–2.

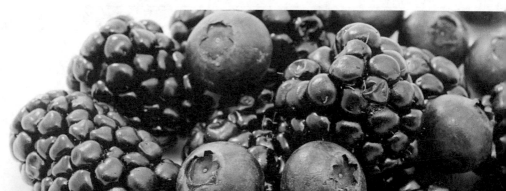

Bladder-Healer Tonic

Cranberry juice has been proven in scientific studies to halt bladder infections. It has substances—tannins and hippuric acid—that prevent bacteria from sticking to the bladder wall. Parsley helps decrease inflammation in the bladder.

2 organic green apples
½ cup cranberries, fresh or thawed if frozen
1 small handful of parsley
1 dark green lettuce leaf
1 small lemon, peeled if not organic

Cut produce to fit your juicer's feed tube. Juice one apple. Turn off the machine, add the cranberries, put the plunger in, turn the machine back on, and juice the berries. Wrap the parsley in the lettuce leaf and juice slowly. Follow with the lemon and second apple. Stir and pour into a glass; drink as soon as possible. Serves 1.

Blood Builder Cocktail

Beets, dandelion leaves, and parsley are all rich in iron and are good tonics for your blood. They are also rich in vitamin C, which works with iron to make it much more absorbable. Dandelion leaves are quite bitter, so don't expect this juice combo to taste yummy. But it's excellent for your body. I usually chase it with water. You could also add a couple drops of stevia to improve the taste.

1 cucumber, peeled if not organic
1 handful of dandelion greens
3–4 carrots, scrubbed well, tops removed, ends trimmed
½ lemon, peeled if not organic

Cut produce to fit your juicer's feed tube. Start by juicing half the cucumber, then add the dandelion greens, followed by the carrots, lemon, and remaining cucumber. Stir the juice and pour into a glass. Drink as soon as possible. Serves 1–2.

Bone Builder

A copper deficiency can result in fragile bones. Carrots, garlic, ginger, and turnips are all rich in copper.

1 handful of parsley
1 kale leaf
1 turnip, scrubbed well

1 lemon, peeled if not organic
4 carrots, scrubbed well, tops removed, ends trimmed
1 garlic clove with peel, washed (optional)

Cut produce to fit your juicer's feed tube. Wrap the parsley in the kale leaf and push through the juicer slowly. Juice all remaining ingredients and stir. Pour into a glass and drink as soon as possible. Serves 1–2.

Brain Helper

Juice up zinc-rich foods such as ginger root, parsley, and carrots. Zinc deficiency has been shown to be a major problem as people age and has been implicated in Alzheimer's disease. People with symptoms of Alzheimer's who receive zinc supplementation have shown improvement in their memory, socialization, and communication.

1 handful of parsley
1 dark green lettuce leaf
3 carrots, scrubbed well, tops removed, ends trimmed
1 apple
2-inch-chunk ginger root

Cut produce to fit your juicer's feed tube place. Wrap the parsley in the lettuce leaf and push through the juicer slowly. Juice all remaining ingredients. Stir and pour into a glass. Drink as soon as possible. Serves 1.

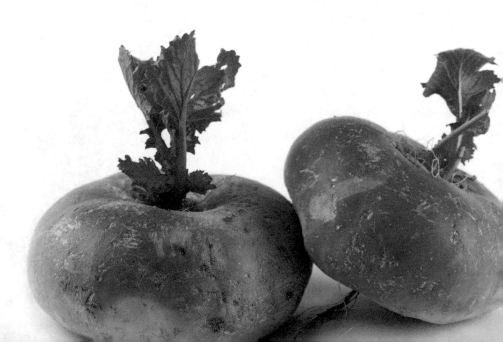

Bruise Mender

If you bruise easily, that is a sign that you're probably deficient in vitamin C. Vitamin C and bioflavonoids work together to help strengthen capillary walls. To improve your intake of vitamin C, be sure to eat foods such as berries, lemon, lime, and dark greens such as kale and parsley.

1 cucumber, peeled if not organic
1 handful of parsley
4 dark green leaves such as collard, chard, or kale
1 cup blueberries (if frozen, thaw first)
1 apple (green is lower in sugar)
1 lemon or lime, peeled if not organic

Cut produce to fit your juicer's feed tube. Juice half of the cucumber. Wrap the parsley in a green leaf and push through the juicer with the other half of the cucumber. Turn off the machine and pour in the berries, then place the plunger on top. Turn the machine back on and push the berries through. Then juice the apple, lemon, and remaining green leaves. Stir the juice and drink as soon as possible. Serves 2.

Calcium Cocktail

Kale and parsley are great sources of very absorbable calcium.

1 handful of parsley
2–3 kale leaves
1 cucumber, peeled if not organic
1 rib of celery with leaves
½ lemon, peeled if not organic
1-inch-chunk ginger root, scrubbed
    or peeled if old

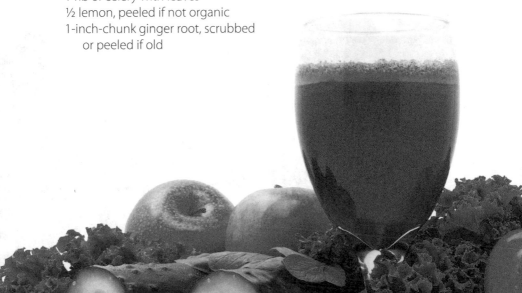

Cut produce to fit your juicer's feed tube. Wrap the parsley in a kale leaf and push through the juicer slowly. Juice all remaining ingredients and stir. Pour into a glass and drink as soon as possible. Serves 1–2.

Cancer-Fighting Tonic

Cruciferous vegetables such as cabbage are known to fight cancer. Cabbage contains a high concentration of indole-3-carbinol and oltipraz—two phytonutrients that help protect and fight against a wide variety of cancers.

¼ small green cabbage (spring or summer cabbage is best)
1 lemon, peeled if not organic
4 ribs of celery with leaves
2 carrots, scrubbed well, tops removed, ends trimmed

Cut produce to fit your juicer's feed tube. Juice ingredients and stir. Pour into a glass and drink as soon as possible. Serves 1.

Cancer-Fighting, Sun-Damage-Blocking Arugula Cocktail

Pound for pound arugula is one of *the most* potent anticancer foods. Some of its phytochemicals, such as glucosinolates and sulforaphanes, are responsible for stimulating enzymes that help the body cleanse away toxins and carcinogens. It also contains carotenes that can protect against sun damage, heart disease, and cancer. In addition, these nutrients improve communication between cells, something that may play a large role in healthy cellular function.

1 cucumber, peeled if not organic
1 handful of arugula
2 ribs of celery with leaves
1-inch-chunk ginger root
1 lemon, peeled if not organic

Cut cucumber in half. Juice half the cucumber. Bunch up arugula and push through juicer with other half of the cucumber followed by celery, ginger, and lemon. Stir the juice and drink as soon as possible. Serves 1.

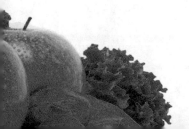

Cholesterol Buster Cocktail

Ginger root has been shown in numerous scientific studies to reduce inflammation. It's inflammation, not cholesterol, that is now implicated in heart disease. But if you are looking to lower your LDL, juice an apple with your ginger root. Apples contain antioxidants that help to halt oxidation of LDL. It is oxidized LDL that is harmful, not regular LDL. Every blood test should distinguish this if it is to be considered reliable.

4 medium carrots, scrubbed well, tops removed, ends trimmed
2 ribs of celery with leaves
2 kale leaves
1 green apple such as Granny Smith or pippin
1-inch-chunk ginger root, scrubbed or peeled if old

Cut produce to fit your juicer's feed tube. Juice ingredients and stir. Pour into a glass and drink as soon as possible. Serves 1–2.

Cold Buster

Grapefruit is loaded with vitamin C and bioflavonoids, especially in the white pithy part. These nutrients support the immune cells. Carrot is rich in beta-carotene, another immune cell superfood. Fresh ginger root is loaded with zinc, which is vital for the immune system. In Chinese medicine ginger root is used for treating colds. Cayenne pepper acts as a decongestant and expectorant. Drink your cold away!

1 grapefruit, peeled
1 carrot, scrubbed well, tops removed, ends trimmed
2–3 kale leaves
1-inch-chunk ginger root
Dash of cayenne pepper

Cut produce to fit your juicer's feed tube. Juice ingredients, add cayenne pepper, and stir. Pour into a glass and drink as soon as possible. Serves 1.

Colon-Cleaning Cocktail

Apples are good sources of soluble fiber, which is very beneficial for the colon.

2 green apples
½ lemon, peeled if not organic
1 handful of spinach
1 handful of parsley
2 dark green lettuce leaves

Cut produce to fit your juicer's feed tube. Juice ingredients and stir. Pour into a glass and drink as soon as possible. Serves 1.

Congestion Helper

In Chinese medicine mustard greens provide what's known as "hot energy," which is good for congestion and poor circulation.

3 carrots, scrubbed well, tops removed, ends trimmed
2 ribs of celery with leaves
2–3 mustard leaves
1 cucumber, peeled if not organic
1 apple (green is lower in sugar)

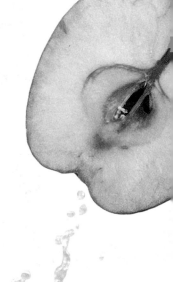

Cut produce to fit your juicer's feed tube. Juice carrots and celery. Roll mustard leaves and place in juicer. Push the greens through with the cucumber and apple. Stir the juice and drink as soon as possible. Serves 1–2.

Constipation Relief

Apples and pears are excellent sources of fiber, which is very beneficial for good colon health.

2 plums, pitted
2 ribs of celery with leaves
1 apple
1 pear
½ cucumber, peeled if not organic

Cut produce to fit your juicer's feed tube. Juice ingredients and stir. Pour into a glass and drink as soon as possible. Serves 2.

THE POWER OF LIVING FOODS

One study surveyed five hundred people on a living foods diet and found that eating a high percentage of live foods helped more than 80 percent of those surveyed lose weight. But this was just the beginning of their health revolution! Respondents also reported a significant improvement in sleep quality and the condition of their skin, hair, nails, and numerous health conditions. The study results also showed a better sense of sight, hearing, smell, and taste on a live foods diet.[1]

Cravings Buster

Sugar and high-carb cravings can be reduced with chromium-rich foods such as apples, parsnips, spinach, carrots, lettuce, string beans, and cabbage.

1 green apple
1 small parsnip
3–4 carrots, scrubbed well, tops removed, ends trimmed
2 dark green lettuce leaves
1 handful of spinach

Cut produce to fit your juicer's feed tube. Juice all ingredients and stir. Pour into a glass and drink as soon as possible. Serves 1–2.

Depression Kicker

Sodium deficiency actually creates symptoms that are a lot like those of depression. But table salt is not a good choice. Use only Celtic sea salt or Himalayan salt. And juice up plenty of sodium-rich vegetables such as celery, chard, beet greens, and spinach.

4 ribs of celery with leaves
1 green apple

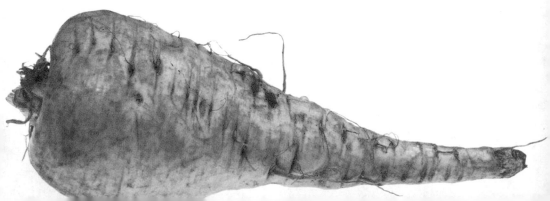

1 medium lemon, peeled if not organic
1 handful of spinach
1–2 chard leaves

Cut produce to fit your juicer's feed tube. Juice all ingredients and stir. Pour into a glass and drink as soon as possible. Serves 1–2.

Digestion Helper

Fennel juice is known to aid digestion and relieve gas. Ginger root is also a gas reliever.

3 fennel stalks with bulb and fronds
1 cucumber, peeled if not organic
1 pear
1-inch-chunk ginger root

Cut produce to fit your juicer's feed tube. Juice all ingredients and stir. Pour into a glass and drink as soon as possible. Serves 1–2.

Diuretic Cocktail

Lemon, parsley, cucumber, and asparagus are all natural diuretics.

1 medium vine-ripened tomato
½ small or medium lemon, washed or peeled if not organic
1 small handful of parsley
1 dark green lettuce leaf
1 cucumber, peeled if not organic
4 asparagus stems

Cut produce to fit your juicer's feed tube. Juice the tomato and lemon. Wrap the parsley in the lettuce leaf and push through the juicer slowly. Follow with the cucumber and asparagus. Stir, pour into a glass, and drink as soon as possible. Serves 1.

Electrolyte Replacer

This is an antioxidant-rich electrolyte replacer that is loaded with vitamin C, bioflavonoids, minerals, and phytonutrients. And it's free of artificial ingredients, sugars, and other undesirable additives that are present in commercial electrolyte replacement drinks.

1 orange, peeled
2 kale, chard, or collard leaves
1 apple
1 lemon, peeled if not organic
1 lime, peeled if not organic
½ tsp. ascorbic acid (vitamin C powder)
¼ tsp. Celtic sea salt

Cut produce to fit your juicer's feed tube. Juice all ingredients, and stir in the ascorbic acid and salt. Pour into glasses and drink as soon as possible. Serves 2.

Fibromyalgia Helper

Apples and cranberries are rich sources of malic acid. People suffering from fibromyalgia pain have shown low muscle-tissue oxygen pressure in affected muscles. Malic acid has been shown to be beneficial in reversing this scenario. Magnesium levels are also low with fibromyalgia, so it's a good idea for fibromyalgia sufferers to include magnesium-rich dark leafy greens in their diets.

1 cup cranberries (thawed if frozen)
1 cucumber, peeled if not organic
3 chard or kale leaves
1 green apple

Cut produce to fit your juicer's feed tube. Turn off juicer and pour in cranberries, then top with plunger. Turn machine back on and juice the berries. Then juice remaining ingredients and stir. Pour into a glass and drink as soon as possible. Serves 1.

Flu Fighter

Garlic is nature's natural antibiotic.

1 handful of watercress or parsley
1 dark green lettuce leaf
1 turnip, scrubbed, ends trimmed (you can include leaves)
3 carrots, scrubbed well, tops removed, ends trimmed
1–2 garlic cloves (no need to peel)
½ lemon, peeled if not organic
½ green apple such as Granny Smith or pippin

Bunch up watercress or parsley and wrap in lettuce leaf. Cut produce to fit your juicer's feed tube. Push lettuce wrap through juicer slowly, and follow with the remaining ingredients. Stir the juice, pour into a glass, and drink as soon as possible. Serves 1.

Folic Acid–Rich Cocktail

Planning on getting pregnant? Folic acid is important to prevent birth defects. Parsnips are rich in folate. This B vitamin also plays a role in reducing heart disease and may help prevent dementia and osteoporosis.

2–3 carrots, scrubbed well, tops removed, ends trimmed
1 cucumber, peeled if not organic
1 small parsnip
1 lemon, peeled if not organic

Cut produce to fit your juicer's feed tube. Juice ingredients and stir. Pour into a glass and drink as soon as possible. Serves 1.

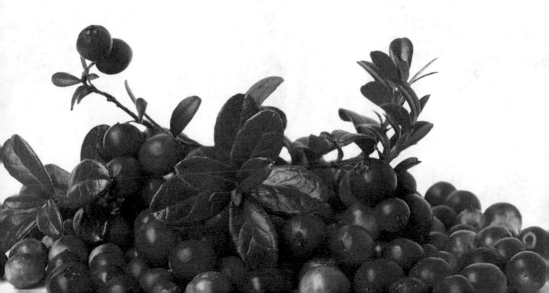

Gallbladder Revitalizer

Purple cabbage, beet with leaves, lemons, apples, and ginger root are all good liver and gallbladder foods because they help to cleanse and support the liver.

3–4 carrots, scrubbed well, tops removed, ends trimmed
½ beet with leaves and stems, scrubbed well
1 lemon, peeled if not organic
½ green apple
¼ purple cabbage
1-inch-chunk ginger root

Cut produce to fit your juicer's feed tube. Juice ingredients and stir. Pour into a glass and drink as soon as possible. Serves 1–2.

Gallstone Solvent Cocktail

Magnesium may help prevent and dissolve gallstones. One way to alleviate a gallbladder attack is to drink a glass of water at the start of the attack. Follow that by taking magnesium, then an hour later drink a bitter liquid such as Swedish bitters and/or a bitter green juice such as dandelion juice. Bitter flavors stimulate bile flow.

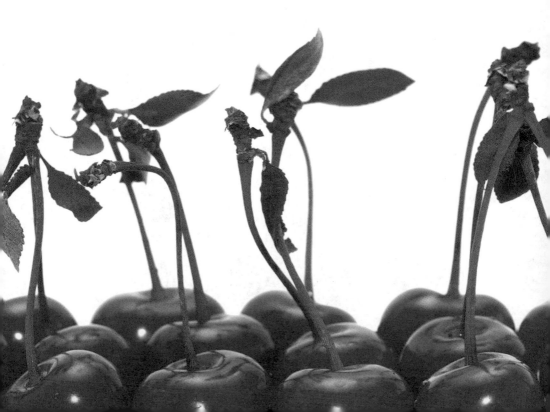

1 green apple (green has less sugar)
3–4 dark leafy greens (rich in magnesium) such as chard or collard greens
1 cucumber, peeled if not organic
1 lemon, peeled if not organic
1 carrot, scrubbed well, tops removed, ends trimmed
Several bitter green leaves such as dandelion, arugula, or mustard

Cut produce to fit your juicer's feed tube. Juice the apple, then roll the green leaves and push through feed tube. Juice remaining ingredients and stir. Pour into a glass and drink as soon as possible. Serves 1.

Good Morning Cocktail

Perk up your morning mood with fennel. Fennel juice has been used as a traditional tonic to help the body release endorphins, the "feel-good" peptides, from the brain into the bloodstream. Endorphins help to diminish anxiety and fear and generate a mood of euphoria.

½ green apple
4–5 carrots, well scrubbed, tops removed, ends trimmed
3 fennel stalks with bulb and fronds
½ cucumber, peeled if not organic
1 handful of spinach
1 dark green lettuce leaf
1-inch-chunk ginger root

Cut produce to fit your juicer's feed tube. Juice all ingredients and stir. Pour into a glass, and drink as soon as possible. Serves 1.

Gout Fighter

Cherries have been shown to reduce the symptoms of gout.

1 green apple
½ pound organic cherries, pits removed
2 ribs of celery with leaves
1 lemon, peeled if not organic

Cut produce to fit your juicer's feed tube. Juice ingredients and stir. Pour into a glass and drink as soon as possible. Serves 1.

Greens and Garlic Yeast Buster

Garlic contains a large number of sulfur-containing compounds that exhibit very potent broad-spectrum antifungal properties.

1 handful of parsley
3 kale leaves
½ medium cucumber, peeled if not organic
1 garlic clove, unpeeled
3 carrots, scrubbed well, tops removed, ends trimmed
2 ribs of celery with leaves

Roll the parsley in the kale leaves and push through the juicer slowly. Juice all remaining ingredients, stir, and pour into a glass. Drink as soon as possible. Serves 1–2.

Happy Liver Cleansing Cocktail

Beets are used traditionally for cleansing the liver. If you have a sugar sensitivity such as diabetes or hypoglycemia, always dilute beet and carrot juice with cucumber and other greens. You may be able to juice only very small portions of beets and carrots if you have sugar metabolism challenges.

3 carrots, scrubbed well, tops removed, ends trimmed
1 cucumber, peeled if not organic
1 beet with stem and leaves, scrubbed well
2 ribs of celery with leaves
1 handful of parsley
1 dark green lettuce leaf
1- to 2-inch-chunk ginger root, scrubbed or peeled if old
½ lemon, peeled if not organic

Cut produce to fit your juicer's feed tube. Juice all ingredients and stir. Pour into a glass and drink as soon as possible. Serves 1–2.

Headache Mender

Cantaloupe and ginger root have been shown to reduce platelet stickiness, which is related to migraine headaches.

½ ripe cantaloupe with seeds, rind removed
½ cucumber, peeled if not organic
1- to 2-inch-chunk ginger root, peeled

Cut produce to fit your juicer's feed tube. Juice all ingredients and stir. Pour into a glass and drink as soon as possible. Serves 1.

Healing Tea

This tea is very good for sore throat, cold, flu, and infections.

2-inch-chunk fresh ginger root, juiced
Juice of ½ medium lemon, peeled if not organic
2 cups purified water
1 Tbsp. loose licorice tea or 1 licorice herbal tea bag (optional)
4–5 whole cloves
1 cinnamon stick, broken
Dash cardamom
Dash nutmeg

Place all ingredients in a saucepan and simmer for about ten minutes. Strain and drink while warm. Serves 1.

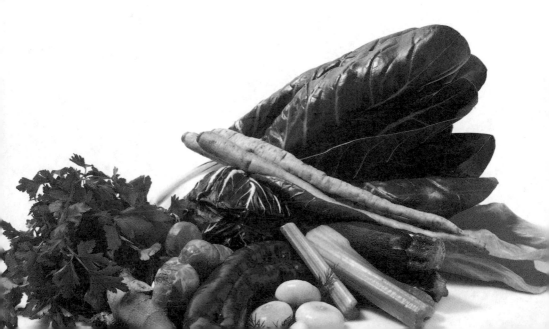

Healthy Bone Solutions

Want to shape up your bones naturally? Include dark leafy greens that are rich in calcium, such as kale, chard, or collard greens. They are also rich in nutrients that work synergistically with calcium such as boron, which prevents loss of calcium; magnesium, which helps calcium get in and out of cells; and vitamin K, which helps anchor calcium in bones.

1 green apple
1 handful of parsley
2–3 kale leaves
1 rib of celery with leaves
1 lemon, peeled if not organic
½- to 1-inch-chunk fresh ginger root, peeled

Cut the apple into sections that fit your juicer's feed tube. Wrap parsley in the kale and push through the juicer slowly. Juice remaining ingredients and stir. Drink as soon as possible. Serves 1.

Hypertension Helper

Beets, carrots, blackberries, cucumber, parsley, celery, broccoli, spinach, and raspberries are all traditional remedies for lowering blood pressure.

1 cucumber, peeled if not organic
3 chard leaves
1 green apple

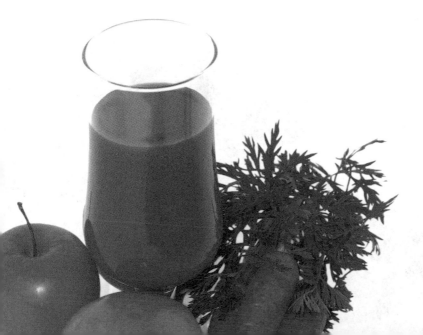

½ beet with leaves
1 cup blackberries or raspberries (thawed if frozen)
½ lemon, peeled if not organic

Cut produce to fit your juicer's feed tube. Juice all ingredients and stir. Pour into a glass and drink as soon as possible. Serves 1.

Immune Support

Studies show that garlic has a natural antibiotic-like effect that is antibacterial, antifungal, anti-parasitic, and antiviral, but it must be consumed raw to have this effect. So juice it up for your immune system.[2]

1 handful of watercress
1 dark green lettuce leaf
5 carrots, scrubbed well, tops removed, ends trimmed
1 green apple
1 large garlic clove with peel
1 cucumber, peeled if not organic

Cut produce to fit your juicer's feed tube. Wrap watercress in lettuce leaf and push through juicer slowly. Juice all remaining ingredients and stir. Pour into glasses and drink as soon as possible. Serves 2.

Immune System Builder

Vitamin C is an important nutrient for the immune system. Include plenty of vegetables and fruit rich in vitamin C, such as kale, parsley, collards, turnip greens, broccoli, watercress, spinach, lemon, and elderberries.

1 handful of parsley or watercress
2–3 kale or collard greens leaves
1 cup elderberries or blueberries
1 green apple
½ cucumber, peeled if not organic
1 lemon, peeled if not organic

Cut produce to fit your juicer's feed tube. Wrap parsley or watercress in the green leaves and push through the juicer slowly with half of the cucumber. Turn off the machine and pour in the berries, then place the plunger on top. Turn the machine on and push the berries through. Juice all remaining ingredients. Stir the juice and drink as soon as possible. Serves 2.

Jet-Lag Helper

Time zone changes are very stressful for the body and especially for the adrenal glands. If you are a frequent traveler, it is very important that you support your adrenals with plenty of organic sodium (celery and cucumber), vitamin C (lemon and parsley), and pantothenic acid (nutritional yeast is the best source).

1 cucumber, peeled if not organic
2 ribs of celery with leaves
1 lemon, peeled if not organic
1-inch-chunk ginger root
½ tsp. ascorbic acid (vitamin C powder)
Sprinkle of nutritional yeast

Cut produce to fit your juicer's feed tube. Juice all ingredients and stir in vitamin C and nutritional yeast. Pour into a glass and drink as soon as possible. Serves 1.

Kidney Tonic

Asparagus is a traditional remedy for bladder and kidney cleansing, and parsley helps to decrease inflammation and irritation in the bladder and urethra. They are also both good diuretics.

1 handful of parsley
1 dark green lettuce leaf
8 asparagus stems
2–3 carrots, scrubbed well, tops removed, ends trimmed
1 cucumber, peeled if not organic
1 medium lemon, washed or peeled if not organic
½ green apple

Cut produce to fit your juicer's feed tube. Wrap parsley in the lettuce leaf and push through the juicer slowly. Juice all remaining ingredients. Pour into a glass, stir, and drink as soon as possible. Serves 1–2.

Liver Tonic

Juice up plenty of liver-friendly foods such as dandelion greens, carrots, and cucumber.

1 handful of dandelion greens
3-4 carrots, scrubbed well, tops removed, ends trimmed
1 cucumber, peeled if not organic
½ lemon, peeled if not organic

Cut produce to fit your juicer's feed tube. Juice all ingredients. Stir the juice, pour into a glass, and drink as soon as possible. Serves 1.

Lung Rejuvenator

Turnip juice has been used as a traditional remedy to strengthen lung tissue.

1 handful of watercress
1 dark green lettuce leaf
1 small turnip, scrubbed well, tops removed,
   ends trimmed
2-inch-thick chunk of jicama, scrubbed
   well or peeled
2–3 carrots, scrubbed well, tops removed,
   ends trimmed
1 garlic clove with peel
½ lemon, peeled if not organic

Bunch up watercress and roll in lettuce leaf; push through juicer slowly. Cut produce to fit your juicer's feed tube. Juice all remaining ingredients. Stir the juice, pour into a glass, and drink as soon as possible. Serves 1.

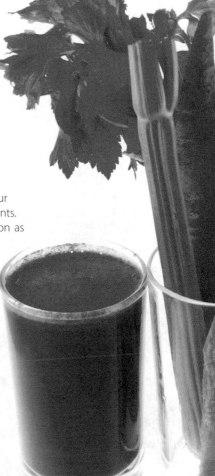

Magnesium Cocktail

The American diet is very low in magnesium. One of magnesium's most important benefits is that it lowers the risk of cardiovascular disease. It's also very helpful for depression, insomnia, and migraines. Juice up plenty of magnesium-rich greens such as beet greens, spinach, chard, collards, parsley, and dandelion greens.

1 handful of parsley
3–4 leaves of chard or collards
3–4 carrots, scrubbed well, tops removed, ends trimmed
2 ribs of celery, with leaves as desired
½ small beet with leaves
1 lemon, peeled if not organic

Cut produce to fit your juicer's feed tube. Wrap parsley in the green leaves and push through the juicer slowly. Juice all remaining ingredients and stir. Pour into a glass and drink as soon as possible. Serves 1.

Memory-Mending Cocktail

Choline is a B vitamin and an important nutrient for brain neurotransmitters, which support memory and intelligence. Juice lots of choline-rich veggies such as green beans, cabbage, spinach, and oranges.

2 medium vine-ripened tomatoes
1 lemon, peeled if not organic
¼ small head green cabbage
8–10 green beans
1 handful of spinach
1 dark green lettuce leaf

Cut produce to fit your juicer's feed tube. Juice ingredients and stir. Pour into a glass and drink as soon as possible. Serves 1–2.

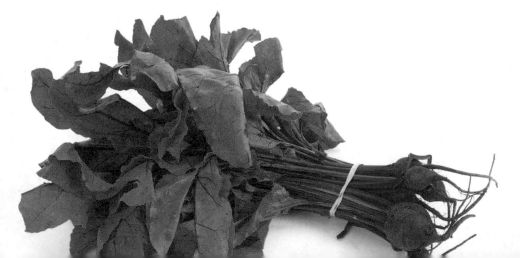

Menopause Helper

Juice up plenty of liver-friendly foods such as beets, celery, carrots, kale, and parsley because the liver is the key organ for hormone metabolism.

1 handful of parsley
2–3 leaves of kale
3 carrots, scrubbed well, tops removed, ends trimmed
2 ribs of celery with leaves
1 cucumber, peeled if not organic
½ beet with leaves
½ green apple
1 lemon, peeled if not organic

Cut produce to fit your juicer's feed tube. Wrap parsley in the kale leaves and push through the juicer slowly. Juice all remaining ingredients and stir. Pour into glasses and drink as soon as possible. Serves 2.

Mood Mender Tonic

Antidepressant use has been linked to thicker arteries, which could contribute to the risk of heart disease and stroke. Raise your endorphins naturally with foods such as fennel. Fennel juice has been used as a traditional remedy to help the body release endorphins into the bloodstream. Endorphins are the "feel-good" peptides from the brain that help to diminish anxiety and fear and generate a mood of euphoria.

3 fennel stalks with bulbs and fronds
3–4 carrots, scrubbed well, tops removed, ends trimmed
2 ribs of celery with leaves
½ pear or ½ apple
½ lemon, peeled if not organic
1-inch-chunk ginger root, peeled

Cut produce to fit your juicer's feed tube. Juice ingredients and stir. Pour into glasses, and drink as soon as possible. Serves 2.

Muscle Beach

3 carrots, scrubbed well, tops removed, ends trimmed
2 cups loosely packed baby spinach
1 cucumber, peeled if not organic
½ green apple

Cut produce to fit your juicer's feed tube. Juice ingredients and stir. Pour into a glass and drink as soon as possible. Serves 1.

Pancreas Rejuvenator

Brussels sprouts and string bean juice have been used as traditional remedies to help strengthen and support the pancreas. Drink this juice recipe before a meal. (If this drink is too strong, dilute with a little water.) For best pancreas support, also avoid refined carbohydrates such as white flour products, sugar of all types, sodas, and all sweets.

2 romaine lettuce leaves
1 cucumber, peeled if not organic
6 string beans
2 brussels sprouts
1 lemon, peeled if not organic
1 large vine-ripened tomato

Cut produce to fit your juicer's feed tube. Tuck the romaine leaves in feed tube and push through with the cucumber. Juice remaining ingredients, finishing with the tomato. Pour into a glass, and drink as soon as possible. Serves 1.

Parasite Kicker

Cabbage and radish are antiparasitic foods.

¼ small head green cabbage
4 ribs of celery with leaves
4 medium carrots, scrubbed well, tops removed, ends trimmed
3 radishes with leaves

Cut produce to fit your juicer's feed tube. Juice ingredients and stir. Pour into a glass, and drink as soon as possible. Serves 1.

Parasite Knockout

Include papaya seeds when juicing papaya. Papaya seeds have been used as a traditional remedy to kill intestinal parasites. One study of Nigerian children who had intestinal parasites found that more than 76 percent of the children were parasite-free after seven days of treatment with papaya seeds. This was compared to only 16.7 percent of the children who received a placebo.[3]

1 papaya with seeds, peeled
½ cucumber, peeled if not organic
2 ribs of celery with leaves
1-inch-chunk ginger root

Cut produce to fit your juicer's feed tube. Juice ingredients and stir. Pour into a glass and drink as soon as possible. Serves 1.

Prostate Helper

Tomato juice has been shown to inhibit the activity of an enzyme that is connected to benign prostate enlargement (BPH).

2 vine-ripened tomatoes
4–5 sprigs of basil
1 large handful of spinach
2 dark green lettuce leaves
1 lemon, peeled if not organic

Juice one tomato. Wrap the basil and spinach in lettuce leaves and push through the machine slowly. Juice all remaining ingredients. Stir the juice, pour in a glass, and drink as soon as possible. Serves 1.

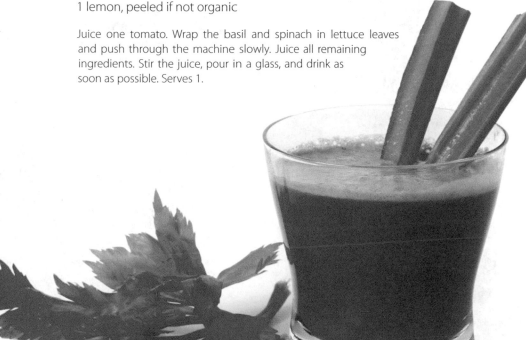

Rheumatoid Arthritis Therapy

Dandelion juice is a traditional remedy for healing rheumatoid arthritis. Drink 1/2 cup in the morning and 1/2 cup in the afternoon to help relieve arthritis pain. Because it is so strong tasting, it's advisable to dilute with other juices or coconut water (my favorite).

1 large bunch dandelion leaves

Juice enough dandelion leaves to make 1/2 cup juice. Dilute with other juice or coconut water as desired. Drink as soon as possible. Serves 1.

Sinus Solution

Radish juice is a traditional remedy to open up the sinuses and support mucous membranes.

2 vine-ripened tomatoes
½ cucumber, peeled if not organic
6 radishes with green leaves
½ lime, peeled if not organic

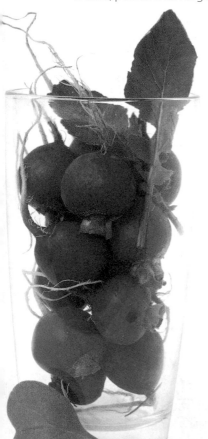

Cut produce to fit your juicer's feed tube. Juice ingredients and stir. Pour into a glass and drink as soon as possible. Serves 1.

Sleep Rejuvenator

Celery has a calming effect, and lettuce is a natural sedative.

2 romaine lettuce leaves
2 ribs of celery with leaves
1 lemon, peeled if not organic
5 medium carrots, scrubbed well, tops
   removed, ends trimmed
4 cauliflower florets, washed

Cut produce to fit your juicer's feed tube. Juice ingredients and stir. Pour into a glass, and drink as soon as possible. Serves 1.

Spring Cocktail

Rejuvenate your system with spring vegetables that cleanse the body from the effects of heavy winter foods. Asparagus is a natural diuretic that helps flush toxins from the body and promotes kidney cleansing.

1 vine-ripened tomato
1 cucumber, peeled if not organic
8 asparagus stems
1 handful of nettles, freshly picked in early spring
1 lemon, peeled if not organic

Cut produce to fit your juicer's feed tube. Juice all ingredients and stir. Pour into a glass, and drink as soon as possible. Serves 1–2.

Sweet Dreaming

Magnesium deficiency may cause you to wake up after a few hours of sleep and not be able to drift off to sleep again. To increase your magnesium intake, juice plenty of magnesium-rich foods such as spinach, parsley, dandelion greens, garlic, blackberries, beets, broccoli, carrots, and celery.

1 small handful of parsley
2 dark green lettuce leaves
1 cup blackberries (thawed if frozen)
3 carrots, scrubbed well, tops removed, ends trimmed
1 handful of spinach
½ cucumber, peeled if not organic
1 rib of celery with leaves

Bunch up the parsley and roll in lettuce leaves. Push through the juicer slowly. Turn off the machine and pour in the berries; then top with plunger. Turn machine back on and push the berries through. Juice all remaining ingredients, stir the juice, and drink as soon as possible. Serves 1.

Sweet Fiber

Pears and apples are good sources of soluble fiber.

1 pear, washed
1 organic apple, any kind, washed

Cut produce to fit your juicer's feed tube. Juice ingredients and stir. Pour into a glass, and drink as soon as possible. Serves 1.

Sweet Regularity

Apples, pears, parsley, and radishes are known to stimulate intestinal motion.

1 apple or 1 pear
1 handful of parsley
1 kale leaf
3–4 radishes with green leaves
½ cucumber, peeled if not organic
1-inch-chunk ginger root

Cut produce to fit your juicer's feed tube. Start with the apple or pear. Wrap the parsley in kale leaf and push through juicer slowly. Juice all remaining ingredients, stir the juice, and drink as soon as possible. Serves 1.

The Rejuvenator

Rejuvenate your body with electrolyte-rich raw juices. Cucumber is particularly hydrating.

2 tomatoes
1 cucumber, peeled if not organic
6–8 string beans
½ lemon or lime, peeled if not organic
Dash of hot sauce

Cut produce to fit your juicer's feed tube. Juice ingredients and stir in hot sauce. Pour into a glass, and drink as soon as possible. Serves 1.

Thyroid-Healing Tonic

Radishes are a traditional tonic for the thyroid.

5 carrots, scrubbed well, tops removed, ends trimmed
½ medium lemon, peeled if not organic
5–6 radishes with tops

Cut produce to fit your juicer's feed tube. Juice ingredients and stir. Pour into a glass, and drink as soon as possible. Serves 1.

Ulcer-Healing Cabbage Cocktail

Scientific research has proven that cabbage juice is an effective treatment for stomach ulcers.[4]

¼ small head green cabbage
3 carrots, scrubbed well, tops removed, ends trimmed
4 ribs of celery with leaves

Cut produce to fit your juicer's feed tube. Juice ingredients and stir. Pour into a glass and drink as soon as possible. Serves 1.

Vision Helper

Carrots are rich in carotenes and are very helpful for strengthening the eyes and improving vision. Blueberries also help improve eyesight, and apples can help remove metals and toxins from the eyes.

3 carrots, scrubbed well, tops removed, ends trimmed
1 cucumber, peeled if not organic
2 kale, chard, or collard leaves
1 cup blueberries, thawed if frozen
½ green apple

Cut produce to fit your juicer's feed tube. Juice the carrots, cucumber, and kale. Turn off the machine and add the blueberries. Top with the plunger. Turn the machine back on and push berries through; then juice the apple. Stir and pour into a glass. Drink as soon as possible. Serves 1.

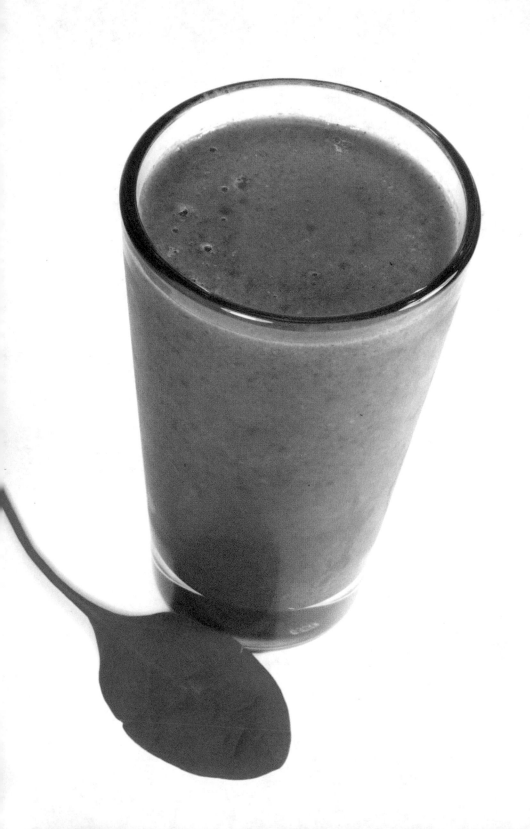

Chapter 8

GREEN SMOOTHIES

GREEN SMOOTHIES MAKE perfect sense for people on the go—not just kids but the whole family. These green drinks can be made in minutes, and you can quickly add a variety of supplements such as vitamin C, barley greens, or bee pollen. You can basically drink your vitamins and minerals on the run! I have created more than one hundred recipes that incorporate greens and taste absolutely yummy. The picky eaters in your family will never even know the greens are there. But the best news is that as you sip your somewhat decadent shake, you'll know you're doing something really good for your body, not just your taste buds.

Acai-Cacao Supreme

1 cup fresh or frozen blueberries
1 cup fresh or frozen raspberries
½ cup plain yogurt
½ cup chopped kale
1 Tbsp. acai powder
1 Tbsp. cacao powder
1–2 drops stevia (optional)

Combine all ingredients in a blender and process well until smooth and creamy. Serve chilled. Serves 2.

HEALTH BENEFITS OF ACAI AND OTHER BERRIES

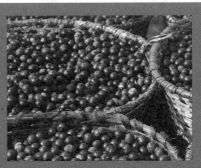

Acai berries are inch-long reddish-purple fruit. They come from the acai palm tree, which is native to Central and South America. Research has examined their antioxidant activity because antioxidants can help prevent diseases caused by oxidative stress, such as heart disease and cancer. Acai berries contain substances known as anthocyanins and flavonoids. Anthocyanins cause the red, purple, and blue shades in many fruits and vegetables. The foods richest in anthocyanins such as blueberries, red grapes, and acai range from deep purple to black. Some studies show that acai has even more antioxidant content than cranberries, raspberries, blackberries, strawberries, and blueberries.[1]

Anthocyanins and flavonoids are potent antioxidants that help defend us against life's stressors. They also have a roll in cell protection by quenching free radicals—harmful products that damage cells. When we include plenty of antioxidant-rich fruits and vegetables in our diets, we slow down the aging process and prevent disease by neutralizing free radicals.

Almond Swirl

1 cup almond milk
2 ripe peaches, pits removed, cut into chunks
½ cup kale, chopped
1–2 drops stevia
1 tsp. pure vanilla extract
½ tsp. pure almond extract
6 ice cubes

Combine all ingredients in a blender and process well until smooth and creamy. Serve chilled. Serves 2.

Amazon Kicker

1 cup fresh apple juice
½ cup frozen unsweetened acai berries
½ cup spinach
1 cup fresh or frozen strawberries
1 medium frozen banana, cut into chunks
4 ice cubes

Combine all ingredients in a blender and process well until smooth and creamy. Serve chilled. Serves 2.

Apple Spice

2 cups plain yogurt
1 cup chopped apple
1 cup baby spinach, packed
½ tsp. ground cinnamon or apple pie spice
½ cup fresh orange juice

Combine all ingredients in a blender and process well until smooth and creamy. Serve chilled. Serves 2.

Avocado Cream

½ cup almond milk
1 avocado, peeled and seeded
1 handful of spinach
2 Tbsp. fresh lemon juice
2–3 drops stevia
1 tsp. pure vanilla extract
1 tsp. organic lemon peel, freshly grated
6 ice cubes

Combine all ingredients in a blender and process well until smooth and creamy. Serve chilled. Serves 1.

Aztec Chili Cacao

1½ cups almond milk
½ cup spinach or chopped kale
1 banana, peeled and cut into chunks
½ vanilla bean
¼ jalapeño pepper, seeds removed unless you like really hot foods
½ tsp. cinnamon
1-2 Tbsp. cacao
Stevia drops to taste
6–8 ice cubes

Combine all ingredients in a blender and process well until smooth and creamy. Serve chilled. Serves 1–2.

Berries 'n' Cream

1 cup strawberries with caps
1 banana, peeled, and cut into chunks
1 cup plain yogurt
½ cup loosely packed flat-leaf parsley
3–4 drops stevia (optional)
6 ice cubes

Combine all ingredients in a blender and process well until smooth and creamy. Serve chilled. Serves 2.

THE ANTI-INFLAMMATORY BENEFITS OF CHILIES

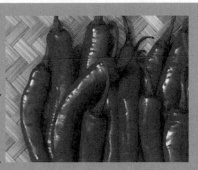

Chili peppers contain a substance known as capsaicin, which gives peppers their spicy taste. Capsaicin inhibits substance P, a neuropeptide associated with inflammation. The hotter the chili pepper, the more capsaicin. The hottest varieties are habañero, and Scotch bonnet jalapeños follow them in intensity. The mildest varieties are Spanish pimientos, Anaheim peppers, and Hungarian cherry peppers.

Capsaicin has been studied as a treatment for arthritis, psoriasis, and diabetic neuropathy. When animals were injected with a substance that causes inflammatory arthritis and were fed capsaicin in their diet, they experienced reduced inflammation and delayed onset of arthritis.[2]

Berry Mania

½ cup almond milk
½ cup plain low-fat yogurt
½ cup chopped kale
½ cup loosely packed baby spinach
½ cup fresh or frozen blueberries
½ cup fresh or frozen raspberries
½ cup fresh or frozen blackberries
1 frozen banana, cut into chunks

Combine all ingredients in a blender and process well until smooth and creamy. Serve immediately. Serves 2.

Berry Smooth

1 cup coconut milk
1 handful of spinach
2 cups fresh or frozen berries (blueberries, blackberries, or raspberries)
6 ice cubes (optional, may not be needed if using frozen fruit)

Combine all ingredients in a blender and process well until smooth and creamy/slushy. Serve as soon as possible. Serves 1.

Berry-Mango-Kale Slushy

1 cup frozen strawberries with caps
1 cup chopped frozen mango
1 cup chopped kale
Juice of 1 lime
4–5 ice cubes

Combine all ingredients in a blender and process well until smooth and creamy/slushy. Serve chilled. Serves 2.

Blueberry Jazz

1 cup almond milk
1½ cup frozen banana cut into chunks (about 2 medium-size bananas)
1½ cups frozen blueberries
½ cup spinach
1–2 Tbsp. fresh lemon juice

Pour the milk into a blender and add the bananas, blueberries, spinach, and lemon juice. Blend until smooth and creamy. Serve as soon as possible. Serves 2.

Body Builder

1 cup almond milk
¼ cup raw cashews
1 cup chopped kale
1 scoop protein powder of choice (whey is best for bodybuilding)
1 Tbsp. pure cold-pressed flaxseed oil
½ tsp. ascorbic acid (vitamin C powder)

3–4 drops liquid stevia
1 frozen banana, cut into chunks

Put all ingredients in a blender and process until smooth and creamy. Serve as soon as possible. Serves 1–2.

Brain Power

½ cup plain yogurt
1 cup fresh or frozen strawberries, with caps
1 cup kale, chopped
½ cup orange juice
1 Tbsp. lecithin granules
1 Tbsp. protein powder of choice
1 tsp. pure vanilla extract
2–3 drops stevia
6–8 ice cubes

Put all ingredients in a blender and process until smooth and creamy. Serve as soon as possible. Serves 1–2.

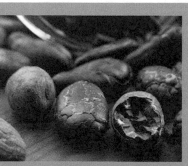

THE ANTIOXIDANT BENEFIT OF CACAO

Cacao beans have been scientifically proven to have high levels of antioxidants. Antioxidants bind up free radicals that cause cellular damage and promote disease. A study published in The Journal of Agricultural and Food Chemistry in 2003 showed that cacao had much higher concentration of antioxidants than other popular sources such as green tea. It has also been shown to have cardiovascular benefits and to protect against cancer.[3]

Cacao Extravaganza

1 cup almond or coconut milk
1 banana, peeled, cut into chunks
1 Tbsp. peanut butter or almond butter
1 Tbsp. cacao powder
½ cup flat-leaf parsley
Sprinkle of cacao nibs on top of smoothie (optional)
6–8 ice cubes

Combine all ingredients in a blender and process well until smooth and creamy. Pour into a glass and sprinkle cacao nibs on top, as desired. Serve chilled. Serves 1.

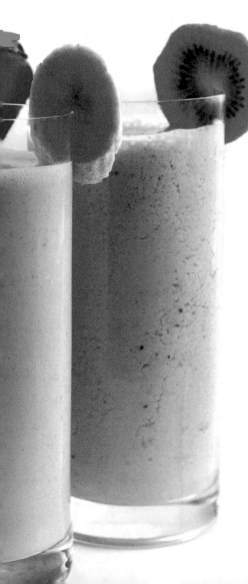

Calcium Booster

Kale is packed with calcium in a form that is assimilated by the body far better than the calcium in dairy products—and that's a great bonus for your bones!

1 cucumber, peeled if not organic
1 cup chopped kale
2 pears (Asian or Bartlett)
1 avocado
6 ice cubes

Chop cucumber, kale, and pear. Place in the blender and process until smooth. Add the avocado and ice, and blend until creamy. Serves 2.

Captain Kidd's Greens

1 cucumber, peeled if not organic
2 ribs of celery
1 handful of parsley or spinach
1 kiwifruit
1 apple
Juice of ½ lemon
6 ice cubes

Chop the cucumber, celery, greens, kiwi, and apple. Place in blender with lemon juice and ice, and process until creamy. Serves 2.

Caribbean Morning

1 cup coconut milk
½ cup fresh orange juice
1 Tbsp. coconut oil
1½ cups fresh or frozen papaya chunks
1 cup fresh or frozen pineapple chunks
½ cup chopped kale
2 Tbsp. unsweetened shredded coconut
6 ice cubes (optional; not needed if using frozen fruit)

Pour the coconut milk, orange juice, and coconut oil in a blender and process until combined. Then add the papaya, pineapple, kale, shredded coconut, and ice cubes; blend again until smooth. Serves 2.

Carnival on Ice

½ cup fresh apple juice (1 apple, juiced)
1 cup fresh or frozen blueberries, rinsed if fresh
1 frozen banana, cut into chunks
1 green leaf lettuce, chopped
½ cup raw cashews
½ tsp. pure vanilla extract
6 ice cubes

Combine all ingredients in a blender and process well until smooth and creamy. Serve chilled. Serves 2.

Carob Classic

1 cup almond or coconut milk
½ cup spinach
2 Tbsp. carob powder (cocoa powder can be substituted)
1 tsp. pure vanilla extract
1 frozen or fresh banana, cut into chunks

Pour the milk into a blender, and add the spinach, carob, vanilla, and banana. Process until smooth and creamy. Pour into a glass and serve as soon as possible. Serves 1.

Chai Green

1 cup almond milk
1 banana, cut into chunks
1 cup chopped greens of choice
½ tsp. ground cinnamon
⅛ tsp. ground cardamom
⅛ tsp. ground coriander
⅛ tsp. ground cloves
⅛ tsp. ground black pepper
5–6 drops stevia or 1 Tbsp. honey
6 ice cubes (or 6 ice cubes of frozen chai green tea)

Combine all ingredients in a blender and process well until smooth and creamy. Serve chilled. Serves 2.

Cherie's Green Morning Blend

½ English cucumber, peeled if not organic and cut into chunks
1 avocado, peeled, seeded, and cut into quarters
1 cup loosely packed baby spinach
Juice of 1 lime
1 Tbsp. green powder of choice (optional)
2–3 Tbsp. ground almonds (optional)

Combine all ingredients in a blender and blend well. Sprinkle ground almonds on top, as desired. Serves 1.

Chia Mia

10 raw almonds
1 Tbsp. raw sunflower seeds
1 Tbsp. chia seeds
1 Tbsp. sesame seeds
1 Tbsp. flaxseeds
1 cup pineapple juice (juice one quarter pineapple, if making fresh)
1 cup chopped parsley
½ cup almond milk
½ tsp. pure vanilla extract
1 Tbsp. protein powder (optional)
6 ice cubes

Place the nuts, seeds, and pineapple juice in a bowl. Cover and soak overnight. Place the nut and seed mixture with the juice in a blender and add the parsley, milk, vanilla, protein powder (if using), and ice cubes. Blend on high speed until smooth. This drink will be a bit chewy because of the nuts and seeds. Serves 2.

Note: To kill molds, add 1/2 tsp. ascorbic acid to juice, then add nuts and soak overnight.

Chocolate Chimps

1 banana, peeled and cut into chunks
1 Tbsp. cocoa or powdered cacao
1 Tbsp. peanut butter or almond butter
½ cup loosely packed baby spinach
½ cup almond milk
1–2 drops stevia
6 ice cubes

Place all ingredients in a blender and process until smooth and creamy. Pour into glasses and serve chilled. Serves 2.

Cocoa Cabana

1 cup almond milk
1½ cups frozen banana, cut into chunks
1 cup chard, chopped
3 Tbsp. unsweetened cocoa powder
½ tsp. cinnamon

Pour the milk into a blender and add the frozen banana chunks, chard, cocoa powder, and cinnamon. Blend until smooth. Serves 2.

Coconut Creamsicle

1 cup coconut milk
1 orange, peeled, cut into chunks
½ cup grated coconut, lightly packed
½ cup loosely packed baby spinach
2 tsp. pure vanilla extract
4–5 drops stevia
6 ice cubes

Place all ingredients in a blender and process until smooth and creamy. Pour into glasses and serve chilled. Serves 2.

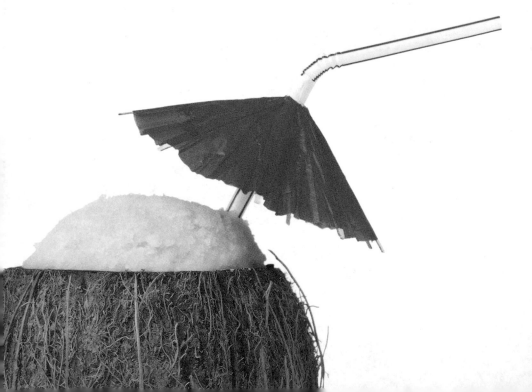

Coconut Green Delight (Yeast-Fat Buster Smoothie)

Coconut oil is an ally in breaking the yeast-fat cycle. One study showed that it was very effective at killing *Candida albicans*.[4] Its medium-chain fatty acids split open the protective outer coating of yeast cells, thus killing the yeast.

1 cucumber, cut into chunks
1 cup raw spinach, kale, or chard, chopped
1 avocado, peeled, seeded, and cut into quarters
½ cup coconut milk
1 Tbsp. organic virgin coconut oil
Juice of 1 lime or lemon

Combine all ingredients in a blender and process until creamy. Serves 2.

Coconut Ice

1 banana, peeled, cut into chunks
1 peach, seed removed
1 cup loosely packed baby spinach
1 cup coconut ice cream

Place all ingredients in a blender and process until smooth and creamy. Pour into a glass and serve chilled. Serves 1.

Columbian Blend

1 cup of coffee or coffee substitute, chilled
1 banana, peeled, cut into chunks
1 Tbsp. powdered cocoa or cacao
½ cup almond milk
½ cup chopped flat-leaf parsley
1–2 drops stevia
6 ice cubes

Place all ingredients in a blender and process until smooth and creamy. Pour into glasses and serve chilled. Serves 2.

Cool Corn Avocado

1 firm-ripe avocado, peeled and seeded
1 garlic clove, chopped
½ tsp. Celtic sea salt
¼ small serrano or jalapeño pepper, stemmed, seeds removed (unless you
    like really hot foods), and coarsely chopped
1 cup almond milk
Juice of 1 lime
1 fresh or frozen ear of corn, shucked, corn cut from cob (optional)

Combine all ingredients except corn kernels in blender and process until smooth
and creamy. Pour into a glass and drink. Or you can pour into bowls, stir in corn
kernels, and eat as a soup. Serve cold. Serves 2.

Cranberry-Cucumber Fat Buster

2 pears, Bartlett or Asian
1 cucumber, peeled if not organic
½ cup loosely packed baby spinach
¼ lemon, peeled if not organic 2 Tbsp. cranberries, fresh or frozen
1-inch-chunk ginger root
6 ice cubes (optional)

Chop up pears and cucumber and blend until smooth. Add lemon juice,
cranberries, ginger, and ice as desired, and blend until creamy. Serves 1.

Dandelion Morning

½ bunch of dandelion greens
2 ribs of celery with leaves
1-inch-chunk fresh ginger root
1 peach, seed removed
1 cup berries, fresh or frozen

Combine all ingredients in a blender and process until smooth and creamy.
Serves 2.

Detox Helper

This smoothie is good for helping detox symptoms or a hangover. The liver is quite adversely impacted by overconsumption of alcohol. Both tomato and lemon juice help to revitalize it and improve vitality. Japanese pickled plums (also known as umeboshi plums, found at health food stores) are used in macrobiotic medicine to counteract the effects of overconsumption of alcohol.

This is because umeboshi is rich in citric acid and phosphoric acid. These organic acids facilitate a rapid breakdown of excess of acids such as lactic acid and pyruvic acid in the body. Such an effect helps eliminate the symptoms of excessively acidic conditions, including a hangover, fatigue, morning sickness, car or seasickness, certain types of headaches, stomach troubles, anemia, and detox symptoms. Umeboshi is also known to stop diarrhea.

1½ cups fresh tomato juice (about 3 tomatoes, juiced)
½ cup fresh carrot juice (3 medium carrots, juiced)
Juice of ½ lemon
½ cup packed baby spinach
2 pickled (umeboshi) plums, seeds removed
6 ice cubes

Place all ingredients in a blender and process until creamy. Serves 2.

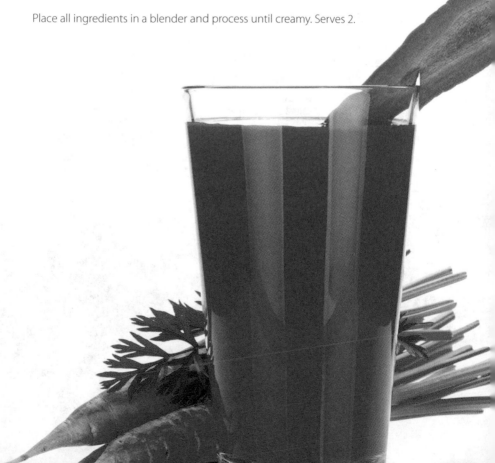

Dilly Sweet Pea

2 cups peas, fresh or frozen (thawed)
3 Tbsp. fresh dill, minced
1 cup purified water (or more as needed)
½ cup fresh lemon juice, peeled if not organic
2 cloves garlic, minced
1–2 tsp. fresh ginger, minced
1½ cups avocado, mashed
½ cup celery with leaves, chopped
¼ tsp. cayenne pepper
3–4 drops liquid stevia
2 tsp. Celtic sea salt or to taste

Combine green peas and dill in a blender with all other ingredients, and process until smooth and creamy. Pour into serving glasses and drink. Or you can pour into bowls, top with 1 Tbsp. dill and additional 1 cup of peas, and serve chilled as a soup. Serves 4.

Dr. Nina's Sweet Dandelion Smoothie

1 pear, Bartlett or Asian
1 apple
1 large handful of dandelion greens
1 cup coconut milk
Juice of ½ lemon, peeled if not organic
¼ cup flaxseeds
6 ice cubes (optional)

Place all ingredients in a blender and process until a creamy and smooth. Serves 2.

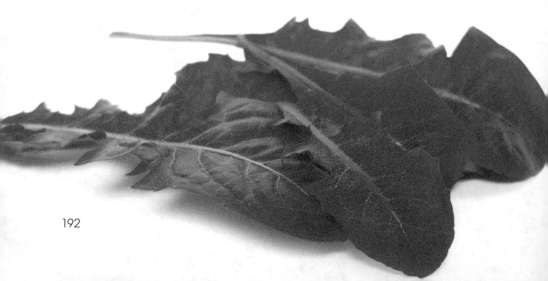

Energy Boost

½ cup fresh carrot juice (3–4 medium carrots, juiced)
½ cup fresh apple juice (about 1½ apples, juiced)
Juice of ½ lemon
½ cup packed baby spinach
½ cup raw cashews
6 ice cubes

Place all ingredients in a blender and process until creamy and smooth. Serves 1.

Fat Burner

Note: Ginger root helps raise metabolism, which helps you burn more calories.

1 cup carrot juice (about 8 carrots)
1 apple, cut into chunks
1 banana, peeled and cut into chunks
1 cup packed baby spinach
1-inch-chunk ginger root
6 ice cubes

Place all ingredients in a blender and process until smooth. Pour into glasses and serve chilled. Serves 2.

Fennel Ice

½ cup fresh fennel juice (½ fennel bulb with fronds)
1 apple, chopped
1 handful of spinach
½ tsp. pure anise extract
¼ cup chopped mint leaves
1 ripe pear, washed, stem removed, and cut into chunks

Pour the fennel juice into a blender; add the apple, spinach, anise, mint, and pear. Blend on high speed until smooth and serve immediately. Serves 2.

Fresh Fig Smoothie

1 cup almond milk
6 fresh ripe figs, cut in half
1 frozen banana, cut into chunks
½ cup loosely packed baby spinach
3 Tbsp. raw cashews
1 tsp. pure vanilla extract
½ tsp. ground nutmeg
6–8 ice cubes

Pour the milk into a blender and add the figs, banana, spinach, cashews, vanilla, nutmeg, and ice cubes as desired. Blend until smooth and serve immediately. Serves 2.

Fruit Salsa Smoothie

1 cup chopped papaya
½ cup chopped mango
¼ cup fresh cilantro, chopped
½ cup fresh orange juice
Juice of 1 lime
½–1 tsp. minced jalapeño pepper without seeds (unless you like really hot foods)
½ tsp. Celtic sea salt

Place all ingredients in a blender and process until smooth. Pour into glasses and serve chilled. Serves 2.

Green Berry Delight

1 cucumber, peeled if not organic
½ apple
1 cup berries (blueberries, raspberries, or blackberries), fresh or thawed if frozen
3–4 dark green leaves (collards, Swiss chard, or kale)
1-inch-chunk ginger root
Juice of ½ lemon, peeled if not organic (Meyers lemons are sweeter)
1 avocado, peeled, seeded, and cut into chunks

Cut the cucumber and apple into chunks. Place the cucumber, berries, and apple in a blender and process until smooth. Chop the greens and ginger and add to the blender along with the lemon juice and avocado. Process until well blended. Serves 2.

Green Creamsicle

1 banana, peeled and cut into chunks
1 cup packed baby spinach
1 cup fresh orange juice
1 cup plain yogurt
6 ice cubes

Combine all ingredients in a blender and process until smooth and creamy. Pour into a glass and serve immediately. Serves 1.

Green Lemon Coconut Ice Cream Shake

½ cup coconut milk
1 cup coconut ice cream
1 cup packed spinach
2 Tbsp. fresh lemon juice
½ tsp. organic lemon peel, freshly
    grated

Combine all ingredients in a blender and process until smooth and creamy. Pour into glasses and serve immediately. Serves 2.

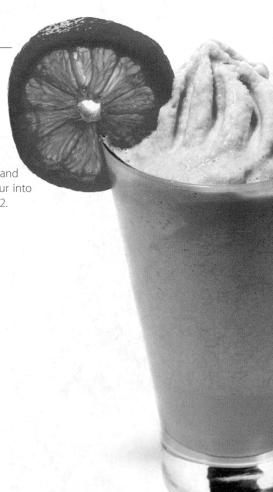

Green Lemonade Slush

2 apples (green is lower in sugar)
Juice of ½ lemon
1 handful of spinach
6–8 ice cubes

Place all ingredients in a blender and process until smooth. Pour into glasses and serve chilled. Serves 2.

SHOULD WE AVOID FOODS HIGH IN OXALATES TO PREVENT KIDNEY STONES?

Oxalates are naturally occurring chemicals that are found in the human body and in animals. But they are most common in fruits and vegetables. As a general rule, the leaves of fruit and vegetables will contain more oxalates than the stems and shoots of the plant. Some health experts encourage people to lightly steam vegetables that are quite high in oxalates. Other pop nutrition experts say we should avoid eating them raw altogether to prevent kidney stones. So what's the real truth of the matter?

A study was published April 2007 in the Journal of the American Society of Nephrology regarding oxalates and kidney stones. It examined the relationship between oxalate intake and nephrolithiasis (kidney stones) in health professionals. Food frequency questionnaires were used to assess oxalate intake every four years. A total of 4,605 incidents of kidney stones were documented over a combined forty-four-year period of follow-up. There was no statistically significant difference in oxalate intake between participants with and without kidney stones.[5]

Studies show a large amount of urinary oxalate is derived from the metabolism of glycine, glycolate, hydroxyproline, and dietary vitamin C. One study showed that a diet high in hydroxyproline (protein from gelatin) increased urinary oxalate excretion by 42 percent.[6] Studies of dietary oxalate and kidney stone risk also must account for other dietary factors such as the intake of magnesium, which may decrease urinary oxalates. The researchers said their data did not support the contention that dietary oxalate is a major risk factor for kidney stones. The risk associated with oxalate intake was modest even in individuals who consumed diets that were relatively low in calcium even though low calcium intake tends to raise the risk of developing kidney stones.

The following foods all contain some form of oxalates:

- Vegetables: celery, collards, dandelion greens, eggplant, green peppers, leeks, okra, parsnips, potatoes, sweet potatoes, pumpkin, rhubarb, rutabagas, spinach, squash (yellow and summer), turnip greens, watercress, and yams

- Fruits: blackberries, blueberries, dewberries, dried figs, gooseberries, raspberries (red and black), grapes (Concord), strawberries, and tangerines

- Herbs and spices: chocolate, ground cinnamon, cocoa, cocoa powder, ginger, lemon peel, lime peel, orange peel, parsley, pepper, pokeweed, sesame seeds, and sorrel

In conclusion, magnesium helps prevent calcium from binding with oxalates and forming kidney stones. The American diet is quite deficient in magnesium. But, interestingly, some of the dark green vegetables (such as chard and spinach) that are particularly high in oxalates are also quite 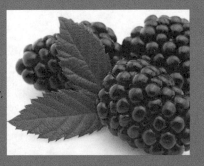 high in magnesium. It looks as though these vegetables came packaged just right.

I don't recommend you avoid eating vegetables raw that are high in oxalates but rather make sure you have enough magnesium in your diet. Foods such as spinach, parsley, dandelion greens, garlic, blackberries, beets, broccoli, carrots, and celery are all rich in magnesium. Include these and other dark leafy greens often in your green smoothies and juices.

Green Mint Dream

1 cup plain yogurt
2 cups cucumber, peeled if not organic and diced
1 handful of spinach
2 Tbsp. scallions, chopped
½ tsp. Celtic sea salt
¼ cup chopped mint leaves
1 garlic clove, peeled and minced

Combine the yogurt with the cucumber, spinach, scallions, salt, mint, and garlic in a blender. Process on high speed until smooth. Pour into glasses and serve immediately. Or you can pour into bowls and serve as a soup. Serves 2.

Green Piña Colada

½ cup coconut milk
1 cup fresh pineapple, peeled if not organic and diced
¼ cup lightly packed grated coconut
1 large handful of spinach
1 tsp. pure vanilla extract
4–5 drops liquid stevia
1 banana, peeled and cut into chunks
6 ice cubes

Pour the milk into a blender and add the pineapple, coconut, spinach, vanilla, stevia, banana, and ice. Blend on high speed until smooth and serve immediately. Serves 2.

Green Power Pro

3 kale leaves, chopped
3 chard leaves, chopped
3 red leaf lettuce leaves, chopped
½ cup parsley, chopped
2 pears, stems removed, cut into chunks
1 banana, peeled and cut into chunks
½ cup almond or coconut milk

Combine all ingredients in a blender and process until smooth and creamy. Pour into glasses and serve immediately. Serves 2.

Green Smoothie Supreme

1 broccoli stem (save the florets for steaming, if you like)
1 apple
1 lemon
½ cucumber, peeled if not organic, cut into chunks
1 handful of spinach
1 small handful of parsley
1 cup blueberries (fresh or frozen)
1 kiwifruit
1 avocado, peeled, seeded, and cut into chunks
2–3 drops stevia
4–6 ice cubes, as desired

Juice the broccoli stem, apple, and lemon. Pour the juice in the blender, and add the cucumber, spinach, parsley, blueberries, kiwi, and avocado. Add stevia if you like it sweeter and ice cubes if you like it cold. Blend until the mixture is smooth and creamy. Serves 2.

Green Tea Freeze

1 cup white grape juice (2 cups green grapes, juiced)
1 ripe medium pear, washed, stem removed, and cut into chunks
1 handful of spinach
1-inch-chunk ginger root
6 green tea ice cubes*

Pour the grape juice into a blender; add the pear, spinach, ginger root, and green tea ice cubes. Blend on high speed until the mixture is smooth and creamy. Serve immediately. Serves 1.

* Note: For green tea ice cubes: Steep one bag of green tea in a cup of hot water for about twenty minutes or until the tea is strong and flavorful. Pour the tea into six ice cube tray squares and freeze.

Greens on the Beach

1 banana, peeled and cut into chunks
1 cup fresh orange juice
3 Tbsp. cocoa or cacao powder
1 cup of your favorite greens, chopped
1 cup plain yogurt
1 tsp. pure vanilla extract
6 ice cubes

Place all ingredients in a blender and process until smooth and creamy. Pour into glasses and serve chilled. Serves 2.

Guava-Pineapple Flip

1 cup coconut milk
1 cup guava nectar
1 cup fresh or frozen pineapple chunks
1 frozen banana, cut into chunks
½ cup loosely packed baby spinach
1 tsp. pure vanilla extract
6 ice cubes (optional, not needed if using frozen fruit)

Combine all ingredients in a blender and process until smooth and creamy. Pour into glasses and serve immediately. Serves 2.

Happy Green Morning

1 cup almond or coconut milk
2 Tbsp. ground flaxseed
2 cups packed baby spinach
½ cup frozen pineapple, chopped
1 frozen banana, cut into chunks

Place all ingredients in a blender and process until smooth and creamy. Pour into glasses and serve chilled. Serves 2.

Happy Road Runner

1 cup blueberries, frozen or fresh
1 banana, peeled, cut into chunks
1 cup chopped kale
1 cup coconut milk
6 ice cubes

Combine all ingredients in a blender and process until smooth and creamy. Pour into glasses and serve chilled. Serves 2.

Hazelnut-Carob Dreamsicle

1 cup almond or hazelnut milk
½ cup hazelnuts
1 frozen banana, cut into chunks
½ cup loosely packed baby spinach
1 Tbsp. carob powder
2–3 drops stevia
6 ice cubes

Combine all ingredients in a blender and process until smooth and creamy. Pour into glasses and serve chilled. Serves 1–2.

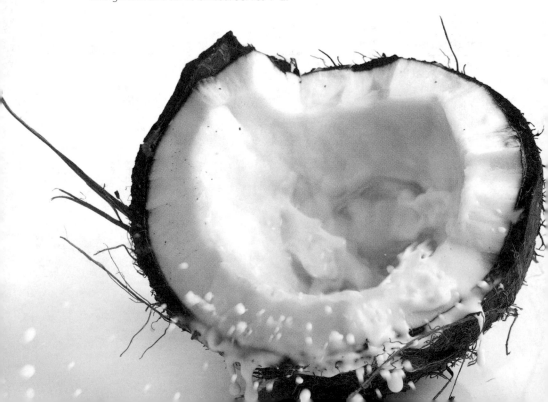

Heavenly Corn-Coriander

4 ears fresh sweet organic corn, shucked and kernels removed
3 cups almond milk
½ cup raw cashews, soaked 1 to 2 hours and drained
¼ cup loosely packed baby spinach
1 garlic clove, peeled
1 small shallot, peeled
2 tsp. Celtic sea salt, or to taste
1 tsp. ground coriander
3–4 drops liquid stevia
1 Tbsp. extra-virgin olive oil
2–3 Tbsp. lime juice or to taste
½ tsp. cayenne pepper

Combine in a blender three-fourths of the corn with almond milk, soaked cashews, spinach, garlic, shallot, salt, coriander, stevia, and olive oil. Puree until smooth, adding water as needed to achieve desired consistency. Add lime juice 1 Tbsp. at a time to taste. Strain to remove any fibers. Stir in cayenne pepper. Pour into glasses and drink. Serves 4.

　　Note: To serve as a soup, blend only three-fourths of the corn with the almond milk; then follow the recipe as directed. Pour into bowls and spoon remaining raw corn kernels into each bowl. Garnish with a dash of ground coriander and a sprig of cilantro, and serve immediately.

Honeydew-Coconut Dream

½ honeydew melon, seeds and rind removed, cut into chunks
1 small handful of mint
1 handful of spinach
1 cup coconut milk
6 ice cubes

Place all ingredients in a blender and process until smooth. Pour into glasses and serve chilled. Serves 2.

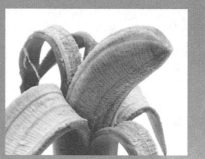

HOW TO FREEZE A BANANA

Always peel the banana before freezing. You can then cut it in chunks and freeze it in a glass container.

Island Breezes

1 ripe mango, peeled, pitted, and cut into chunks
1 banana, cut into chunks
½ cup coconut milk
½ cup green leaf lettuce, chopped
¾ cup pomegranate seeds
6 ice cubes

Place all ingredients in a blender and process until smooth and creamy. Pour into a glass and serve chilled. Serves 1.

Java Jive

1 cup coffee or coffee substitute, chilled
1 banana, peeled and cut into chunks
1 Tbsp. powdered cocoa or cacao
1 Tbsp. peanut butter or almond butter
½ cup almond milk
½ cup loosely packed baby spinach
1–2 drops stevia
6 ice cubes

Combine all ingredients in a blender and process until smooth and creamy. Pour into glasses and serve immediately. Serves 2.

Just Peachy Slushy

1 cup plain yogurt
2 peaches, seed removed, cut into chunks, frozen
½ cup loosely packed baby spinach
6–8 ice cubes

Place all ingredients in a blender and process until smooth and creamy. Pour into a glass and serve chilled. Serves 1.

Leapin' Leprechauns

1 cup fresh apple juice (about 2 apples juiced)
1 frozen banana, cut into chunks
1 cup chopped greens such as kale, chard, or collards
6–8 ice cubes

Place all ingredients in a blender and process until smooth and creamy. Pour into glasses and serve chilled. Serves 2.

Mango Acai

1 cup almond or coconut milk
1 cup acai juice
1½ cups chopped mango
½ cup loosely packed baby spinach
1 frozen banana, cut into chunks
3–4 ice cubes

Combine all ingredients in a blender and process until smooth and creamy. Pour into glasses and serve chilled. Serves 2.

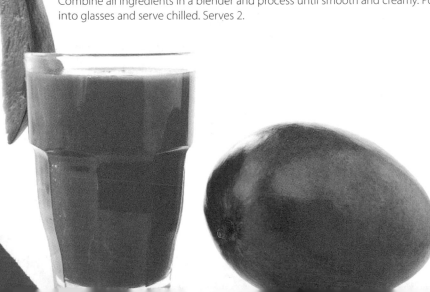

Mango in Paris

2 kale leaves
1 mango, peeled and seeded
1 peach, seeded and cut into chunks
1 banana, cut into chunks
1 cup plain yogurt
6 ice cubes

Combine all ingredients in a blender and process until smooth. Pour into glasses and serve chilled. Serves 2.

Mediterranean Medley

1 cup purple grapes
1 banana, cut into chunks
1 cup packed baby spinach
Juice of 1 lemon
6 ice cubes

Place all ingredients in a blender and process until smooth. Pour into glasses and serve chilled. Serves 2.

Mercury Cleansing Smoothie

Cilantro is known to help the body detox from mercury.

1 handful of cilantro
1 cup chopped fresh parsley
1 rib of celery with leaves, chopped
1 mango or 1 papaya, peeled and seeded, cut into chunks
Juice of 1 lemon
½ cup fresh apple juice
2 cups chopped stinging nettles (optional)

Combine all ingredients in a blender and process until smooth and creamy. Pour into glasses and serve immediately. Serves 2.

Middle Eastern Bliss

1 cup fresh apple juice (about 2 apples juiced)
½ cup plain low-fat yogurt
½ cup loosely packed baby spinach
5 small fresh, ripe black figs, cut in half
½ tsp. pure almond extract
¼ tsp. ground cloves
6 ice cubes

Combine all ingredients in a blender and process until smooth. Pour into glasses and serve chilled. Serves 2.

Minted Mango Sparkler

1 small handful of fresh mint leaves
1 lime, juiced
2 mangoes, peeled and seeded, cut into chunks
1 cup sparkling water, chilled

Combine mint, lime juice, and mango chunks in blender; puree. Pour into glasses and stir in the sparkling water. Serve chilled. Serves 2.

Muscle Power

Cashews and chard are rich in magnesium, which plays a critical role in converting carbohydrates to energy. Magnesium is needed for cells to make ATP—the body's energy fuel. This mineral also controls heartbeat and muscle contractions, and it is important for muscle relaxation and prevention of muscle spasms.

⅔ cup fresh apple juice (about 2 apples, juiced)
1 cup fresh or frozen strawberries
½ cup raw cashews
1 cup chopped chard
1 Tbsp. protein powder of choice
½ tsp. ascorbic acid (vitamin C powder)
6 ice cubes

Pour the apple juice into a blender and add the strawberries, cashews, chard, protein powder, ascorbic acid, and ice. Blend on high speed until smooth; serve immediately. Serves 1.

Nightcap

½ cup almond milk
2 Tbsp. tahini (sesame butter)
1½ tsp. organic orange peel, freshly grated
1 Tbsp. lecithin granules
1 tsp. pure vanilla extract
1 banana, peeled and cut into chunks
2 kale leaves, chopped
½ orange, peeled and cut into chunks
4–6 ice cubes

Combine all ingredients in a blender and process until smooth and creamy. Pour into a glass and serve chilled. Serves 1.

On the Green

1 cucumber, peeled if not organic and chopped
½ cup chopped kale
½ cup chopped parsley
½ cup frozen pineapple chunks
1 Tbsp. organic virgin coconut oil
6–8 ice cubes

Combine all ingredients in a blender and process until smooth and creamy. Pour into a glass and serve chilled. Serves 1.

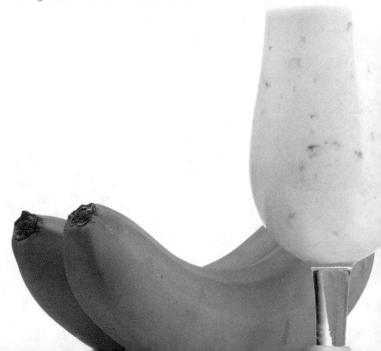

Orange-Vanilla-Kale Shake

Juice of 2 oranges
2 kale leaves, chopped
1 cup plain yogurt
½ tsp. pure vanilla extract
⅛ tsp. orange-flower water (available at specialty food shops and some
    supermarkets; optional)
6–8 ice cubes

Combine all ingredients in a blender and process until smooth and creamy. Pour
into a glass and serve chilled. Serves 1.

Papaya Dreamsicle

1 cup almond milk
1 papaya, cut into chunks and frozen (about 1½ cups)
½ cup chopped flat-leaf parsley
1½ tsp. organic lemon peel, freshly grated
1 tsp. pure vanilla extract

Place all ingredients in a blender and process until smooth and creamy. Pour into
glasses and serve chilled. Serves 1–2.

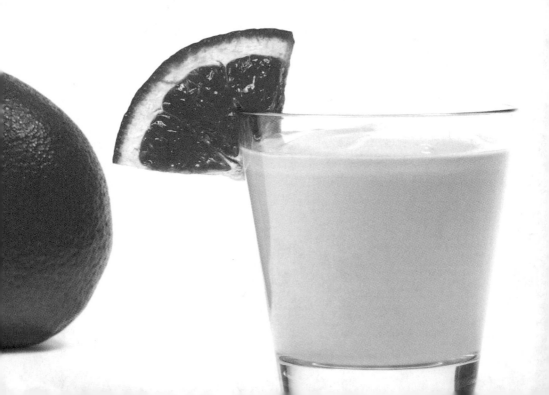

Peach-Almond Breeze

½ cup fresh orange juice
½ cup almond milk
2 peaches, pits removed
1 cup loosely packed baby spinach
1 frozen banana, cut into chunks
¼ cup almonds, toasted
6–8 ice cubes

Place all ingredients in a blender and process until smooth and creamy. Pour into glasses and serve chilled. Serves 1–2.

Peaches and Spice

¾ cup apple juice (about ½ large apple, juiced)
½ cup plain yogurt
1½ cups fresh or frozen peaches, cut into chunks
½ cup spinach
1 frozen banana, cut into chunks
1 tsp. cinnamon
3–4 ice cubes (optional, not needed if using frozen fruit)

Pour the juice into a blender; add the yogurt, peaches, spinach, banana, cinnamon, and ice as needed. Blend until smooth and creamy. Serves 2.

Peanut Butter Mania

1 cup strawberries with caps
1 banana, cut into chunks
1 cup packed baby spinach
3 Tbsp. peanut butter
6 ice cubes

Place all ingredients in a blender and blend until smooth. Pour into glasses and serve chilled. Serves 2.

Pecan Holiday

1 cup fresh pineapple juice
½ cup pineapple chunks
1 frozen banana, cut into chunks
1 cup packed baby spinach
¼ cup pecans
6–8 ice cubes

Combine all ingredients in a blender and blend until smooth. Pour into glasses and serve chilled. Serves 2.

Peppermint Pattie

1 cup fresh apple juice
1 ripe pear, stem removed, cut into chunks
1 kiwifruit, peeled and cut into chunks
1 handful of spinach
¼ cup chopped mint
4–5 drops stevia
⅛ tsp. pure peppermint extract
6 peppermint tea ice cubes*

Pour the apple juice into a blender; add the pear, kiwi, spinach, mint leaves, stevia, peppermint extract, and peppermint tea ice cubes. Blend on high speed until smooth and creamy. Serve immediately. Serves 2.

   * Note: For peppermint tea ice cubes: Steep one peppermint herbal tea bag in a cup of hot water for about twenty minutes or until the tea is strong and flavorful. Pour the tea into six ice cube tray squares and freeze.

Pineapple Mania

1 cup pineapple, peeled if not organic and chopped
1 cup strawberries with caps
1 papaya, peeled (a few seeds may be used)
1 cup baby spinach
6 ice cubes

Place all ingredients in a blender and process until smooth. Pour into glasses and serve chilled. Serves 2.

Pineapple-Mint Frosty

1 cup fresh pineapple juice
1½ cups frozen pineapple chunks
1 cup packed baby spinach leaves
½ cup mint, chopped
4 ice cubes

Combine all ingredients in a blender and process until smooth. Pour into a glass and serve chilled. Serves 1.

Plum Delicious

½ cup almond milk
1 tsp. pure vanilla extract
5 purple plums, rinsed, seeds removed,
    cut in half
1 frozen banana, cut into chunks
½ cup loosely packed baby spinach
6 ice cubes

Combine the milk in a blender with the vanilla, plums, banana, spinach, and ice. Blend on high speed until smooth and creamy; serve immediately. Serves 1.

Razzmatazz

1 cup fresh orange juice
1 banana, peeled, cut into chunks
1 cup loosely packed baby spinach
½ cup raspberries, fresh or frozen
½ cup blueberries, fresh or frozen
½ cup blackberries, fresh or frozen
3 ice cubes if using frozen fruit; 6 ice
    cubes if using fresh fruit

Place all ingredients in a blender and process until smooth. Pour into glasses and serve chilled. Serves 2.

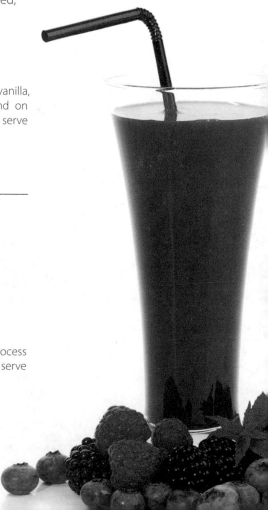

Rhubarb-Banana Flip

2 stalks rhubarb, no leaves (they are toxic), cut into chunks
1 frozen banana, cut into chunks
1 cup almond milk
1 tsp. cinnamon
1 handful of spinach
1–2 drops stevia
6 ice cubes

Combine all ingredients in a blender and process until smooth. Pour into glasses and serve chilled. Serves 2.

Rockin' Berries

1 cup almond or coconut milk
2 cups fresh or frozen berries (blueberries, blackberries, or raspberries)
½ cup acai berry juice
1 cup baby spinach
1 tsp. pure vanilla extract
6 ice cubes (optional, may not be needed if using frozen fruit)

Combine the milk in a blender with the berries, juice, vanilla, and ice. Blend until smooth and creamy. Serves 1.

Sail Away

1 papaya, peeled and cut into chunks (about 1½ cups); you may use a few seeds
1 cup packed baby spinach
¾ cup coconut milk
¼ cup grated unsweetened coconut, lightly packed
1½ tsp. organic lime peel, freshly grated
1 tsp. pure vanilla extract

Combine all ingredients in a blender and process until smooth and creamy. Serve immediately. Serves 1–2.

Savory Tomato

6–8 medium tomatoes
Juice of 1 lemon
1 avocado, peeled, seeded, cut into chunks
⅔ cup of sunflower or buckwheat sprouts
½ cup packed baby spinach
¼ cup fresh basil, chopped
1 small clove garlic, chopped
Pinch Celtic sea salt or dash of Braggs Liquid Amino Acids

Chop tomatoes and puree in a blender. The puree should be somewhat chunky. Then add lemon juice, avocado, sprouts, spinach, basil, garlic, and salt or liquid amino acids. Blend and pour into glasses. Or you can pour into bowls and serve as soup. Serves 2.

Southwestern Green Smoothie

1-¼ cups fresh carrot juice (5–7 medium carrots, or approximately 1 pound, yields about 1 cup)
1 handful of spinach
1 avocado, peeled and seeded, cut into chunks
½ tsp. ground cumin

Combine all ingredients in a blender and process until smooth. Serve chilled. Serves 1.

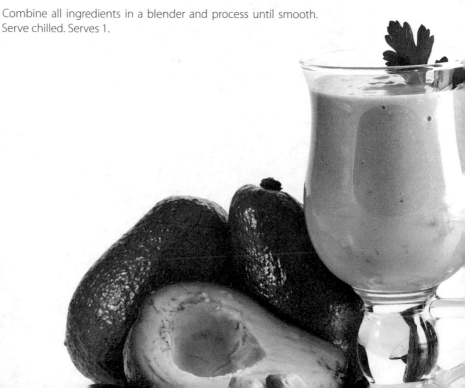

Spice Girl

1 cup fresh green apple juice (about two apples)
1 banana, peeled and cut into chunks
1-inch-chunk ginger root (juice with the apples or grate)
4 oz. soft silken organic tofu
½ cup packed baby spinach
½ tsp. cinnamon
⅛ tsp. ground black pepper
⅛ tsp. ground cumin
⅛ tsp. ground cardamom

Combine all ingredients in a blender and process until smooth and creamy. Pour into glasses and serve chilled. Serves 2.

Spicy Tomato

5 tomatoes, chopped
1 cucumber, peeled if not organic
3 ribs of celery, cut into chunks
1 kale leaf, chopped
1 garlic clove, peeled and chopped
Dash of kelp powder or dulse flakes
1 avocado, peeled, seeded, and cut into chunks

Combine tomatoes in blender and process on low. Add cucumber and continue to blend on low; then add celery and blend on high quickly. Add a bit of water if mixture becomes too thick. Next add kale leaf, garlic, and kelp or dulse, and blend mixture on high. Add avocado and blend on high until well mixed. Serves 2.

Spring Blossom

1 cup fresh orange juice (2 medium oranges, juiced)
½ cup flat-leaf parsley, chopped
½ cup plain low-fat yogurt
1 tsp. orange-blossom water
1 tsp. grated organic orange peel
6 ice cubes

Combine all ingredients in a blender and process until smooth and creamy. Pour into a glass and serve chilled. Serves 1.

Sprouted Almond-Vanilla Smoothie

1 cup raw almonds
1 cup unsweetened almond milk
1 cup berries of choice
1 cup chopped greens, such as kale, collards, or chard
½ tsp. pure vanilla extract
6 ice cubes

Soak almonds in purified water overnight so they will sprout. (Sprouting allows the almond to partially germinate, which removes the enzyme inhibitors and increases nutrient value.) Blend together almonds, almond milk, berries, vanilla, and ice. Pour into glasses and serve as soon as possible. Serves 2.

Strawberry Coconut Cream

½ cup almond milk
5 oz. soft silken organic tofu
⅓ cup grated coconut, lightly packed
8–10 strawberries, fresh or frozen
½ cup loosely packed baby spinach
1 tsp. pure vanilla extract
6 ice cubes

Place all ingredients in blender and process until creamy and smooth. Serve chilled. Serves 2.

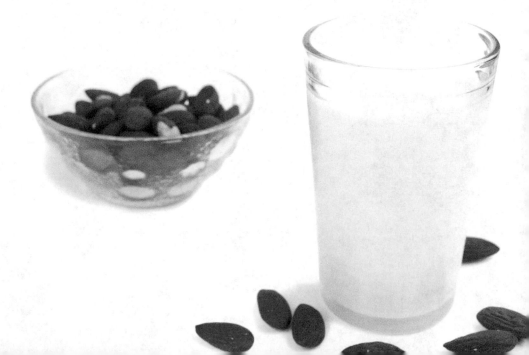

Strawberry Shangri-La

1 quart strawberries with caps
1 ripe banana, cut into chunks
1 handful of spinach
½ cup silken organic tofu
½ cup fresh orange juice
6–8 ice cubes

Combine all ingredients in a blender and process until smooth. Pour into glasses and serve cold. Serves 2.

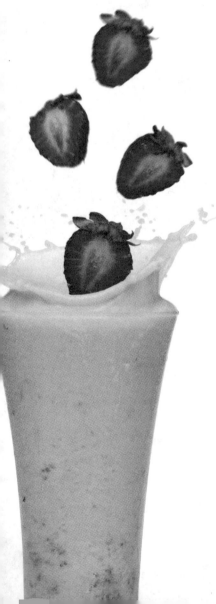

Summer Blueberry Breeze

1 frozen banana, cut into chunks
½ cup fresh or frozen blueberries
1 romaine lettuce leaf, chopped
1 small handful of mint, chopped
6 ice cubes

Combine all ingredients in blender and process until smooth. Serve chilled. Serves 1.

Sunday Brunch

2 tomatoes, chopped
1 handful of cilantro, chopped
Juice of 1 lime
Pinch of Celtic sea salt
Dash of hot sauce

Combine all ingredients in blender and process until well combined. Serve chilled. Serves 2.

Super Savory Green Smoothie

1-¼ cups fresh cucumber juice (about 1 large or 2 medium cucumbers, peeled if not organic)
2 ribs of celery with leaves, juiced
1 kale leaf, chopped
1 avocado, peeled, seeded, and cut into chunks
1 garlic clove, peeled
4 oz. soft silken organic tofu
½ cup flat-leaf parsley, coarsely chopped
2 tsp. sweet onion, minced
1 tsp. dried dill weed

Pour the cucumber and celery juices into a blender; add the kale, avocado, garlic, tofu, parsley, onion, and dill. Blend on high speed until smooth and creamy; serve immediately as it does not taste good if it sits. Serves 2.

Sweet Green Tahini

1 apple, washed and juiced (about ½ cup juice)
1 rib of celery with leaves, juiced
1 Tbsp. tahini (sesame butter)
1 banana, peeled and cut into chunks
½ cup packed baby spinach
6 ice cubes

Combine all ingredients in blender and process until creamy and smooth. Serve chilled. Serves 1.

Tahini Green Smoothie

1 cup plain yogurt
1 large handful of spinach
1 kale leaf, chopped
1 Tbsp. tahini (sesame butter)
1 tsp. pure raspberry extract
1 tsp. pure vanilla extract
½ tsp. organic orange peel, freshly grated
1–2 drops stevia (optional)
6 ice cubes

Place all ingredients in blender and process until creamy and smooth. Serve chilled. Serves 1.

Thai Green Smoothie

1 mango, peeled, stone removed, and cut into chunks
1 orange, peeled and cut into chunks
1 handful of spinach
½ banana, peeled and cut into chunks
1-inch-chunk lemongrass, bruised
½ cup coconut milk
6 ice cubes

Place all ingredients in blender and process until creamy and smooth. Serve chilled. Serves 2.

Tomato-Lemon Twister

1 cup tomato juice (2–3 medium tomatoes, juiced)
2 tomatoes, cut into chunks and frozen
½ cup packed baby spinach
Juice of 1 lemon
1 tsp. organic lemon rind, freshly grated
6 fresh basil leaves, rinsed

Pour the tomato juice into a blender and add the frozen tomato chunks, spinach, lemon juice, lemon rind, and basil. Blend on high speed until smooth. Serve immediately. Serves 2.

Tomato-Lemon-Cucumber Smoothie

2 tomatoes, cut into chunks
1 cucumber, peeled if not organic, cut into chunks
Juice of 1 lemon
1 handful of cilantro
1 avocado, peeled and seeded, cut into chunks

Place all ingredients in a blender and process until smooth. Pour into glasses and serve chilled. Serves 2.

Top of the Mornin'

½ cup almond milk
1 cup plain low-fat yogurt
1 cup frozen peaches in chunks
1 cup frozen blueberries
½ cup packed baby spinach
4–5 drops stevia
1 tsp. pure vanilla extract
Ground almonds or chia seeds for garnish (optional)

Place all ingredients in a blender and process until smooth and creamy. Pour into glasses, sprinkle ground almonds or chia seeds on top as desired, and serve chilled. Serves 2.

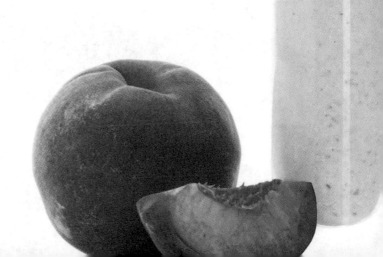

Tropical Frosty

1 cup fresh pineapple, peeled if not organic and chopped
1 orange, torn into segments
1 frozen banana, cut into chunks
1 cup fresh strawberries with caps
1 cup packed baby spinach
Juice of 1 lemon
Juice of 1 orange
6–8 ice cubes

Place all ingredients in a blender and process until smooth. Pour into glasses and serve chilled. Serves 2.

Tropical Green Smoothie

2 kale leaves, chopped
1 papaya, peeled and chopped (you can use a few seeds)
1 ripe mango, peeled, pitted, and chopped
1 handful of spinach
Juice of 1 lime
1 tsp. fresh ginger, peeled and chopped
1 cup coconut milk
6–8 ice cubes

Place all ingredients in a blender and process until smooth. Pour into glasses and serve chilled. Serves 2.

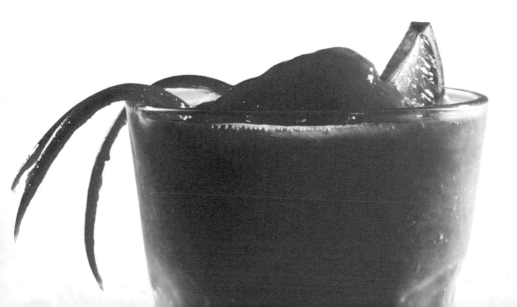

Tropical Treat

¾ cup coconut milk

1 papaya, peeled, seeds removed, cut into chunks, and frozen (makes about 1½ cups)

1½ tsp. organic orange peel, freshly grated

1 tsp. pure vanilla extract

1 cup baby spinach

Pour the milk into a blender, then add the papaya, orange peel, vanilla, and spinach. Blend on high speed until smooth and serve immediately. Serves 2.

Tip: To freeze papaya, simply place the papaya chunks in a freezer bag and freeze them until solid.

Viva La Berries

1 banana, peeled and cut into chunks

1 cup plain yogurt

½ cup blueberries, fresh or frozen

½ cup strawberries, fresh or frozen

½ tsp. pure vanilla extract

3–6 ice cubes, depending on whether you're using fresh or frozen fruit

Place all ingredients in a blender and process until smooth. Pour into glasses and serve chilled. Serves 2.

Weight-Loss Partner

1 cup coconut milk

1 cup berries of choice

½ cup packed baby spinach

1–2 Tbsp. protein powder of choice

1 Tbsp. organic virgin coconut oil

1 Tbsp. ground flaxseeds

1 tsp. pure vanilla extract

¼ tsp. almond extract

2–3 drops stevia

6–8 ice cubes

Combine all ingredients except ice in a blender, and process until creamy and smooth. Add ice after the coconut oil is blended so that it won't clump. You may use more or less ice, depending on how cold you like your smoothie. Serves 1–2.

Workout Buddy

½ cup almond milk
½ cup soft silken organic tofu
1 banana, peeled and cut into chunks
1 handful of spinach
2 Tbsp. peanut butter or almond butter
1 Tbsp. flaxseed
1 tsp. pure vanilla extract
1 tsp. wheat germ
½ tsp. ascorbic acid (vitamin C powder)
1 scoop protein powder of choice
3–4 drops liquid stevia
6 ice cubes

Place all ingredients in a blender and process until creamy and smooth. Drink as soon as possible. Serves 1–2.

Yam Dream

1½ cups yam juice (about 2 large yams)
1 cup almond, oat, or rice milk
½ cup packed baby spinach
¼ cup red onion, chopped
1 avocado, peeled, seeded, and cut into chunks
1 tsp. nutmeg
¼ tsp. cinnamon
¼ tsp. ground allspice
¼ tsp. ground mace
¼ tsp. cardamom

Juice about two large yams to yield about 1½ cup of yam juice. Let the juice sit in a large measuring cup or bowl until the starch settles to the bottom. It will look thick and white. This should take about an hour. Pour off the clear juice but not the starch, as this will make it gritty. Pour the yam juice and milk in a blender. Add the spinach, onion, and avocado; blend until smooth. Add the spices and blend until combined. Pour into glasses and serve. Or you can pour into bowls and serve as soup. Serves 2.

THE JUICE LADY'S BIG BOOK OF JUICES AND GREEN SMOOTHIES SHOPPING GUIDE

P EOPLE HAVE ASKED me many times to provide a shopping guide to help them get started juicing. Below is a basic list to get you to the supermarket, farmer's market, or local grocer and home again with some essential ingredients to begin making juice. This list should provide enough produce for one person to juice for about a week. Be sure to check out the recipes before you shop so you can add the specific items you'll need to make the recipes you want to try.

- 5–10 pounds organic carrots
- 7 lemons or limes; or 3 or 4 of each
- 7 cucumbers
- 1 bunch celery
- 2 bunches chard or collard greens
- 1 bunch parsley
- 1 big ginger root
- 7 apples (green are lower in sugar)

Appendix B

THE JUICE LADY'S BIG BOOK OF JUICES AND GREEN SMOOTHIES RESOURCE GUIDE

SIGN UP FOR the Juice Lady's free Juice Newsletter at www
.juiceladyinfo.com.

Cherie's websites

- www.juiceladyinfo.com—information on juicing and weight loss
- www.cheriecalbom.com
- www.sleepawaythepounds.com—information about the Sleep Away the Pounds program and products
- www.gococonuts.com—information about the Coconut Diet and coconut oil

The Juice Lady's health and wellness juice retreats

I invite you to join us for a week that can change your life! Our retreats offer gourmet organic raw foods with a three-day juice fast midweek. We offer interesting, informative classes in a beautiful, peaceful setting where you can experience healing and restoration of body and soul. For more information, a brochure, and dates for the retreats, call 866-843-8935.

Schedule a nutrition consultation with the Juice Lady

Call 866-843-8935.

Schedule the Juice Lady to speak for your organization

Call 866-843-8935.

Other books by Cherie and John Calbom

These books can be ordered at any of the websites above or by calling 866-8GETWEL (866-843-8935).

- Cherie Calbom, *The Juice Lady's Weekend Weight-Loss Diet* (Siloam)
- Cherie Calbom, *The Juice Lady's Living Foods Revolution* (Siloam)
- Cherie Calbom, *The Juice Lady's Turbo Diet* (Siloam)
- Cherie Calbom, *The Juice Lady's Guide to Juicing for Health* (Avery)
- Cherie Calbom and John Calbom, *Sleep Away the Pounds* (Wellness Central)
- Cherie Calbom, *The Wrinkle Cleanse* (Avery)
- Cherie Calbom and John Calbom, *The Coconut Diet* (Wellness Central)
- Cherie Calbom, John Calbom, and Michael Mahaffey, *The Complete Cancer Cleanse* (Thomas Nelson)
- Cherie Calbom, *The Ultimate Smoothie Book* (Wellness Central)

Juicers

Find out about the best juicers recommended by Cherie. Call 866-8GETWEL (866-843-8935) or visit www.juiceladyinfo.com.

Dehydrators

Find out the best dehydrators recommended by Cherie. Call 866-8GETWEL (866-843-8935) or visit www.juiceladyinfo.com.

Lymphasizer

To view the Swing Machine (lymphasizer), visit www.juiceladyinfo .com or call 866-8GETWEL (866-843-8935).

Veggie powders

To purchase or get information on Barley Max, Carrot Juice Max, and Beet Max powders, go to www.juiceladyinfo.com or call 866-8GETWEL (866-843-8935). (These powders are ideal for when you travel or when you can't get juice.)

Virgin coconut oil

For more information on virgin coconut oil, go to www .juiceladyinfo.com and www.gococonuts.com, or call 866-8GETWEL (866-843-8935). To save money, order larger sizes such as gallons or quarts, which you won't typically find in the stores.

Supplements

- Multivitamins by Thorne Research: call 866-843-8935.

- Digestive enzymes Ness Formula #4 and #16 are excellent to aid digestion. Taken between meals, they help clean up undigested proteins. With the addition of enzymes, you should notice that your hair and nails grow better. Call 866-8GETWEL (866-843-8935).

- Calcium Citrate or Calcium Citramate (contains both calcium citrate-malate and malic acid; offers good solubility and superb absorption when compared to other forms of calcium) by Thorne Research: call 866-843-8935.

- Magnesium Citrate or Magnesium Citramate (as magnesium citrate-malate and malic acid) by Thorne Research: call 866-843-8935.

- Vitamin C with bioflavonoids or Buffered C Powder (contains ascorbic acid, calcium, magnesium, and potassium) by Thorne Research or Allergy Research: call 866-843-8935.

- Vitamin D₃ (1,000 or 5,000 mg) by Thorne Research: call 866-843-8935.

Colon cleanse products

Call 866-843-8935 for more information on Cherie's fiber recommendations below.

- Medibulk by Thorne (psyllium powder, prune powder, apple pectin)

- Colon Cleanse Kit: After years of eating standard food, it's quite common to build up a layer of mucoid plaque—hardened mucuslike material and food residue that can coat the gastrointestinal tract. Nutrients are absorbed through the intestinal wall. The plaque hinders our ability to absorb nutrients, which can lead to numerous health problems. This colon cleanse kit contains products that can pull the plaque from your intestinal wall and carry it out of your system—Digestive Stimulator, Toxin Absorber, glass shaker jar, and user guide and dosage calendar. Specify ginger or peppermint flavor. For more information, visit www.juiceladyinfo.com.

Internal cleansing kit

The complete and comprehensive internal cleansing kit contains eighteen items for a twenty-one-day cleanse program. You get a free colon cleanse kit, along with Liver-Gallbladder Rejuvenator, Friendly Bacteria Replenisher, Parasite Cleanser, Lung Rejuvenator, Kidney and Bladder Rejuvenator, Blood and Skin Rejuvenator, and Lymph

Rejuvenator, along with glass shaker jar and user guide and dosage calendar. Specify ginger or peppermint flavor. Cost $279, less 5 percent discount.

You may order the cleansing products and get the 5 percent discount by calling 866-843-8935. If you want to read more about the cleansing kits, go to my website www.juiceladyinfo.com. You will need to order via the toll-free number to get the discount, however. Mention my special book discount price.

Candida albicans cleanse products

- Total Body Internal Cleanse Kit—visit the website www .juiceladyinfo.com or call 866-843-8935.

Heavy metal and toxic compounds cleanse products

For all these products, visit www.juiceladyinfo.com or call 866-843-8935.

- MetalloClear—designed to help patients stay healthy by providing specialized support for heavy metal metabolism
- Heavy Metal Support by Thorne—replaces important minerals and other nutrients lost during metal chelating

Kidney cleanse herbs

- Kidney & Bladder Rejuvenator—visit the website www .juiceladyinfo.com or call 866-843-8935.

Liver/gallbladder cleanse products

For all these products, visit www.juiceladyinfo.com or call 866-843-8935.

- Detox Nutrients Packet (Liver Cleanse)—complete supplement "take-anywhere" packets for detoxification support
- Chinese herbal tinctures (4-part kit) to use with Cherie's Liver Detox Program

Lung rejuvenator

Visit www.juiceladyinfo.com or call 866-843-8935.

Lymph rejuvenator

Visit www.juiceladyinfo.com or call 866-843-8935.

Parasite cleanse products

For all these products, visit www.juiceladyinfo.com or call 866-843-8935.

- Large Para Cleanser 1 and 2 and Small Para Cleanser
- Total Body Internal Cleanse Kit (includes Para Cleanse Kit and a free colon cleanse kit)

Skin and blood rejuvenator

Visit www.juiceladyinfo.com or call 866-843-8935.

Information and Products for Specific Disorders

Sleep disorders

Testing neurotransmitters is the best way to determine if you have depletion in brain chemicals that could be causing sleep problems. Testing can be completed whether you are taking medications or not. You can determine if your neurotransmitters are out of balance by taking the Brain Wellness Programs Self Test. Just go to www.neurogistics.com and click "Get Started." Use the practitioner code SLEEP (all caps). You can order the program, which includes a urine in-home test that will yield a report on your neurotransmitter levels.

You'll be given a customized protocol with guidelines for the right amino acids for you to take to help correct your imbalances. Or you can call 866-843-8935 for more information.

NOTES

Chapter 1
All About Juicing

1. PCC Sound Consumer, "Light Affects Nutrients," March 2012, http://www.pccnaturalmarkets.com/sc/1203/light_nutrients.html (accessed July 30, 2012).

2. Hong Wang, Guohua Cao, and Ronald L. Prior, "Total Antioxidant Capacity of Fruits," *Journal of Agricultural and Food Chemistry* 44, no. 3 (March 19, 1996): 701–705.

3. Renu Gandhi and Suzanne M. Snedeker, "Consumer Concerns About Pesticides in Food," Fact Sheet #24, Program on Breast Cancer and Environmental Risk Factors, Cornell University, March 1999.

4. D. Winchester, J. Huskins, and J. Ying, "Agrichemicals in Surface Water and Birth Defects in the United States," *Acta Paediatrica* (Oslo, Norway) 98, no. 4 (1992): 664–669.

5. A. Ascherio, H. Chen, M. G. Weisskopf, et al., "Pesticide Exposure and Risk for Parkinson's Disease," *Annals of Neurology* 60, no. 2 (2006): 197–203.

6. L. A. McCauley, W. K. Anger, M. Keifer, R. Langley, M. G. Robson, and D. Rohlman, "Studying Health Outcomes in Farmworker Populations Exposed to Pesticides," *Environmental Health Perspectives* 114, no. 3 (2006): 953–960.

7. Jon Ungoed-Thomas, "Official: Organic Really Is Better," *Sunday Times*, October 28, 2007, viewed at http://www.longnaturalhealth.com/health-articles/organic-food-vs-inorganic-food (accessed July 30, 2012).

8. Virginia Worthington, "Nutritional Quality of Organic Versus Conventional Fruits, Vegetables, and Grains," *Journal of Alternative and Complementary Medicine* 7, no. 2 (April 2001): 161–173.

9. Tara Parker-Pope, "Five Easy Ways to Go Organic," *New York Times*, October 22, 2007, http://well.blogs.nytimes.com/2007/10/22/five-easy-ways-to-go-organic/ (accessed July 30, 2012).

10. Ibid.

11. Bob Williams, "Produce Treated With Pesticides Not Limited to Grocery Stores," *Fergus Falls Journal*, August 8, 2007, http://www.ewg

.org/news/produce-treated-pesticides-not-limited-grocery-stores (accessed July 31, 2012).

12. Marilynn Preston, "Stay Away From the Dirty Dozen," HeraldTribune .com, May 25, 2012, http://www.heraldtribune.com/article/20120529/ ARCHIVES/205291003 (accessed July 31, 2012); Environmental Working Group, "EWG's 2012 Shopper's Guide to Pesticides in Produce," http://www.ewg.org/foodnews/summary/ (accessed July 31, 2012).

13. George L. Tritsch, "'Nuked Food'—the Dangers of Irradiated Food," TrueHealth.org, http://www.truehealth.org/nukedfood.html (accessed February 5, 2010).

14. G. Löfroth, "Toxic Effects of Irradiated Foods," *Nature 211* 302 (July 16, 1966): abstract viewed at http://www.nature.com/nature/journal/ v211/n5046/pdf/211302a0.pdf (accessed July 31, 2012).

15. Environmental Working Group, "EWG's 2012 Shopper's Guide to Pesticides in Produce."

16. J. S. de Vendômois, F. Roullier, D. Cellier, and G. E. Séralini, "A Comparison of the Effects of Three GM Corn Varieties on Mammalian Health," *International Journal of Biological Sciences* 5, no. 7 (2009): 706–726, http://www.biolsci.org/v05p0706.htm (accessed July 25, 2012).

17. David Derbyshire, "Fears Grow as Study Shows Genetically Modified Crops 'Can Cause Liver and Kidney Damage,'" DailyMail.co.uk, January 21, 2010, http://www.dailymail.co.uk/news/article-1244824/Fears-grow -study-shows-genetically-modified-crops-cause-liver-kidney-damage.html (accessed July 31, 2012).

18. de Vendômois, Roullier, Cellier, and Séralini, "A Comparison of the Effects of Three GM Corn Varieties on Mammalian Health."

19. James E. McWilliams, "The Green Monster," Slate.com, January 28, 2009, http://www.slate.com/articles/health_and_science/green_ room/2009/01/the_green_monster.html (accessed July 31, 2012).

20. United States Food and Drug Administration, "Regulation of Foods Derived From Plants," statement of Lester M. Crawford before the Subcommittee on Conservation, Rural Development, and Research House Committee on Agriculture, June 17, 2003, http://www.fda .gov/NewsEvents/Testimony/ucm161037.htm (accessed July 31, 2012).

21. Deborah B. Whitman, "Genetically Modified Foods: Harmful or Helpful?" CSA Discovery Guide, April 2000, http://www.csa.com/ discoveryguides/gmfood/overview.php (accessed July 31, 2012).

22. Ibid.

23. Emma Young, "GM Pea Causes Allergic Damage in Mice," NewScientist.com, November 21, 2005, http://www.newscientist.com/article/dn8347 (accessed July 31, 2012).

24. Mavis Butcher, "Genetically Modified Food—GM Foods List and Information," Disabled-World.com, September 22, 2009, http://www.disabled-world.com/fitness/gm-foods.php (accessed July 31, 2012).

25. Joseph Mercola, "First-Ever Lifetime Feeding Study Finds Genetically Engineered Corn Causes Massive Tumors, Organ Damage, and Early Death," Mercola.com, September 22, 2012, http://articles.mercola.com/sites/articles/archive/2012/09/22/superbugs-destruct-food-supply.aspx (accessed October 11, 2012).

26. Ibid.

Chapter 2
Simple Juice Recipes

1. ScienceDaily.com, "Blueberries May Help Reduce Belly Fat, Diabetes Risk," April 20, 2009, http://www.sciencedaily.com/releases/2009/04/090419170112.htm (accessed October 23, 2012).

2. Niki Fears, "Cranberries and Weight Loss," eHow.com, http://www.ehow.com/about_5417851_cranberries-weight-loss.html (accessed October 23, 2012).

3. Tom Marshall, "Arsenic in Apple Juice: How Much Is Too Much?", *Tampa Bay Times*, March 14, 2010, http://www.tampabay.com/news/health/article1079395.ece (accessed July 31, 2012).

4. Jason Roberge, Andrew T. Abalos, Julia M. Skinner, Mike Kopplin, and Robin B. Harris, "Presence of Arsenic in Commercial Beverages," *American Journal of Environmental Sciences* 5, no. 6 (December 31, 2009): 688–694.

5. NBC25 Newsroom, "Dr. Oz Finds Arsenic in Many Apple Juice Brands," September 15, 2011, http://www.minbcnews.com/news/story.aspx?id=663511 (accessed July 31, 2012).

6. Marshall, "Arsenic in Apple Juice: How Much Is Too Much?"

7. Ibid.

8. Timothy J. A. Key, Margaret Thorogood, Paul N. Appleby, and Michael L. Burr, "Dietary Habits and Mortality in 11,000 Vegetarians and Health Conscious People: Results of a 17-Year Follow-Up," *British Medical Journal* 313 (September 28, 1996): 775.

Chapter 3
Gourmet and Exotic Juice Blends

1. ScienceDaily.com, "Brain Chemical Boosts Body Heat, Aids in Calorie Burn, UT Southwestern Research Suggests," July 7, 2010, http://www.sciencedaily.com/releases/2010/07/100706123015.htm (accessed July 31, 2012).

2. Ibid.

3. Angeline Oppenheimer, "Raw Garlic for Weight Loss," eHow.com, http://www.ehow.com/way_5243593_raw-garlic-weight-loss.html#ixzz19dMcUepI (accessed July 31, 2012).

4. Amy Chan and Thomas B. Shea, "Dietary Supplementation With Apple Juice Decreases Endogenous Amyloid-β Levels in Murine Brain," *Journal of Alzheimer's Disease* 16, no. 1 (January 2009): 167–171, viewed at http://iospress.metapress.com/content/y57409g28gvm0v0h/fulltext.pdf (accessed July 31, 2012).

Chapter 4
Green Juice Recipes

1. R. Akilen, A. Tsiami, D. Devendra, and N. Robinson, "Glycated Haemoglobin and Blood Pressure-Lowering Effect of Cinnamon in Multi-Ethnic Type 2 Diabetic Patients in the UK: A Randomized, Placebo-Controlled, Double-Blind Clinical Trial," *Diabetic Medicine* 27, no. 10 (October 2010): 1159–1167, http://onlinelibrary.wiley.com/doi/10.1111/j.1464-5491.2010.03079.x/full (accessed August 1, 2012).

2. Pat Crocker, "Spring Bitters: From Dandelion to Radicchio—Mean Greens Are the Taste of the Season," *Vitality*, http://vitalitymagazine.com/food-features/spring-bitters (accessed August 2, 2012).

Chapter 7
Juice Remedies and Rejuvenators

1. Lenka J. Zajic, "Raw Food Diet Study," *The Iowa Source*, August 2006, http://www.iowasource.com/food/lenkastudy_0806.html (accessed August 3, 2012).

2. Adam Cloe, "How Much Garlic Equals an Antibiotic?", LiveStrong.com, July 10, 2011, http://www.livestrong.com/article/489317-how-much-garlic-equals-an-antibiotic/ (accessed August 28, 2012).

3. HealthyBodyDaily.com, "Dr. Oz: Parasites—Symptoms and Warning Signs of Parasites and How to Get Rid of Them," http://healthybodydaily.com/dr-oz-in-case-you-missed-it/dr-oz-parasites-symptoms-and-warning-signs-of-parasites-and-how-to-get-rid-of-them (accessed August 3, 2012); "Protect Yourself From Parasites," *The Dr. Oz Show*, March 14, 2012, http://www.youtube.com/watch?v=yRglUAttmzQ (accessed July 24, 2012).

4. Don Amerman, "Benefits and Side Effects of Cabbage Juice," LiveStrong.com, August 7, 2011, http://www.livestrong.com/article/510151-benefits-and-side-effects-of-cabbage-juice/ (accessed August 28, 2012).

Chapter 8
Green Smoothies

1. WedMD.com, "Acai Berries and Acai Berry Juice—What Are the Health Benefits?", June 23, 2012, http://www.webmd.com/diet/guide/acai-berries-and-acai-berry-juice-what-are-the-health-benefits (accessed August 3, 2012).

2. WHFoods.com, "Chili Pepper, Dried," http://www.whfoods.com/genpage.php?tname=foodspice&dbid=29 (accessed August 3, 2012).

3. Robert Shifko, "Health Benefits of Cacao Beans," LiveStrong.com, December 10, 2010, http://www.livestrong.com/article/330290-health-benefits-of-cacao-beans (accessed August 3, 2012).

4. Agalee Jacob, "Candida Diet and Coconut Milk," LiveStrong.com, January 14, 2011, http://www.livestrong.com/article/356535-candida-diet-coconut-milk (accessed August 3, 2012); D. O. Ogbolu, A. A. Oni, O. A. Daini, and A. P. Oloko, "In Vitro Antimicrobial Properties of Coconut Oil on Candida Species in Ibadan, Nigeria," *Journal of Medical Food* 10, no. 2 (June 2007): 384–387, http://www.ncbi.nlm.nih.gov/pubmed/17651080 (accessed August 3, 2012).

5. Eric Taylor and Gary Curhan, "Oxalate Intake and the Risk for Nephrolithiasis," *Journal of the American Society of Nephrology* 18, no. 7 (May 30, 2007): 2198–2204, http://jasn.asnjournals.org/content/18/7/2198.full (accessed August 3, 2012).

6. Ibid.

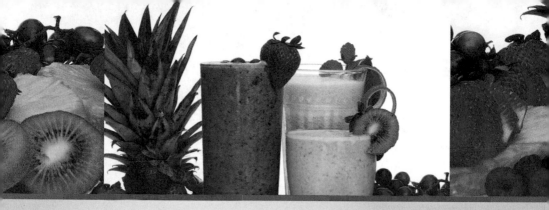

A lifestyle plan that will help you become

HEALTHIER AND HAPPIER FOR LIFE!

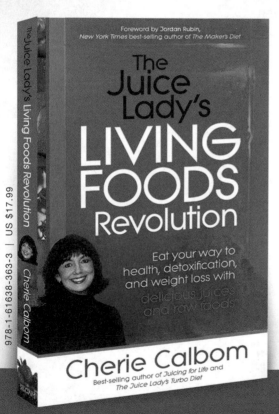

Foreword by Jordan Rubin,
New York Times best-selling author of *The Maker's Diet*

The
Juice
Lady's
LIVING
FOODS
Revolution

Eat your way to
health, detoxification,
and weight loss with
delicious juices
and raw foods

Cherie Calbom
Best-selling author of *Juicing for Life* and
The Juice Lady's Turbo Diet

978-1-61638-363-3 | US $17.99

The Juice Lady's Living Foods Revolution   Cherie Calbom

Nutrition expert Cherie
Calbom shows you how
to enjoy the benefits of
adding more live, raw
foods to your diet.

- Detoxify and Lose Weight
- Slow the Aging Process
- Conquer Adrenal Fatigue
- Boost Your Immune System

SILOAM
11249A

AVAILABLE WHEREVER CHRISTIAN BOOKS ARE SOLD
www.CharismaHouse.com   www.facebook.com/CharismaHouse

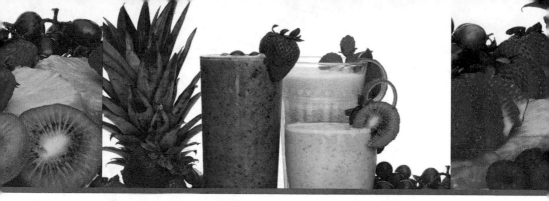
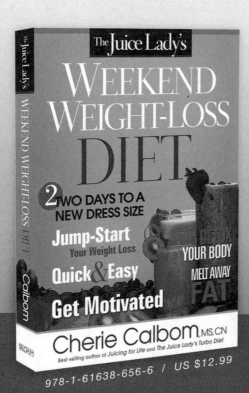
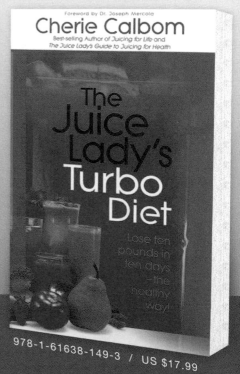

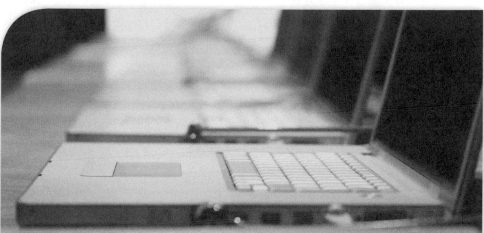

FREE NEWSLETTERS
TO HELP EMPOWER YOUR LIFE

Why subscribe today?

❏ **DELIVERED DIRECTLY TO YOU.** All you have to do is open your inbox and read.

❏ **EXCLUSIVE CONTENT.** We cover the news overlooked by the mainstream press.

❏ **STAY CURRENT.** Find the latest court rulings, revivals, and cultural trends.

❏ **UPDATE OTHERS.** Easy to forward to friends and family with the click of your mouse.

CHOOSE THE E-NEWSLETTER THAT INTERESTS YOU MOST:

- Christian news
- Daily devotionals
- Spiritual empowerment
- And much, much more

SIGN UP AT: **http://freenewsletters.charismamag.com**

6178